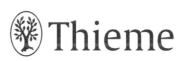

Surgical Care of the Painful Degenerative Lumbar Spine

Evaluation, Decision-Making, Techniques

Edgar N. Weaver, Jr., MD
Vice Section Chief
Neurosurgery
Virginia Tech Carilion School of Medicine
Roanoke, Virginia, USA

with

James B. Macon, MD
Neurosurgeon
Future NeuroSpine, Inc.
Wellesley, Massachusetts, USA

Lydia Prokosch
Medical Illustrator
Floyd, Virginia, USA

75 illustrations

Thieme
New York • Stuttgart • Delhi • Rio de Janeiro

Executive Editor: Timothy Hiscock
Managing Editor: Nikole Y. Connors
Director, Editorial Services: Mary Jo Casey
Production Editor: Torsten Scheihagen
International Production Director: Andreas Schabert
Editorial Director: Sue Hodgson
International Marketing Director: Fiona Henderson
International Sales Director: Louisa Turrell
Director of Instutional Sales: Adam Bernacki
Senior Vice President and Chief Operating Officer:
    Sarah Vanderbilt
President: Brian D. Scanlan
Medical illustrator: Lydia Prokosch
Printer: King Printing

Library of Congress Cataloging-in-Publication Data

Names: Weaver, Edgar N., Jr., author.
Title: Surgical care of the painful degenerative lumbar spine :
evaluation, decision-making, techniques / Edgar N. Weaver, Jr.
Description: First edition. | New York : Thieme, [2018] |
Includes bibliographical references and index.
Identifiers: LCCN 2017059649 (print) | LCCN 2017061060
(ebook) | ISBN 9781626238077 (e-book) | ISBN
9781626238060 (print) | ISBN 9781626238077 (ebook)
Subjects: | MESH: Lumbar Vertebrae–surgery | Interverte-
bral Disc Displacement–surgery | Low Back Pain–surgery
Classification: LCC RD771.B217 (ebook) | LCC RD771.B217
(print) | NLM WE 750 | DDC 617.5/64–dc23
LC record available at https://lccn.loc.gov/2017059649

Important note: Medicine is an ever-changing science undergoing continual development. Research and clinical experience are continually expanding our knowledge, in particular our knowledge of proper treatment and drug therapy. Insofar as this book mentions any dosage or application, readers may rest assured that the authors, editors, and publishers have made every effort to ensure that such references are in accordance with **the state of knowledge at the time of production of the book**.

Nevertheless, this does not involve, imply, or express any guarantee or responsibility on the part of the publishers in respect to any dosage instructions and forms of applications stated in the book. **Every user is requested to examine carefully** the manufacturers' leaflets accompanying each drug and to check, if necessary in consultation with a physician or specialist, whether the dosage schedules mentioned therein or the contraindications stated by the manufacturers differ from the statements made in the present book. Such examination is particularly important with drugs that are either rarely used or have been newly released on the market. Every dosage schedule or every form of application used is entirely at the user's own risk and responsibility. The authors and publishers request every user to report to the publishers any discrepancies or inaccuracies noticed. If errors in this work are found after publication, errata will be posted at www.thieme.com on the product description page.

Some of the product names, patents, and registered designs referred to in this book are in fact registered trademarks or proprietary names even though specific reference to this fact is not always made in the text. Therefore, the appearance of a name without designation as proprietary is not to be construed as a representation by the publisher that it is in the public domain.

Thieme Publishers New York
333 Seventh Avenue, New York, NY 10001 USA
+1 800 782 3488, customerservice@thieme.com

Thieme Publishers Stuttgart
Rüdigerstrasse 14, 70469 Stuttgart, Germany
+49 [0]711 8931 421, customerservice@thieme.de

Thieme Publishers Delhi
A-12, Second Floor, Sector-2, Noida-201301
Uttar Pradesh, India
+91 120 45 566 00, customerservice@thieme.in

Thieme Publishers Rio de Janeiro, Thieme Publicações Ltda.
Edifício Rodolpho de Paoli, 25º andar
Av. Nilo Peçanha, 50 – Sala 2508,
Rio de Janeiro 20020-906 Brasil
+55 21 3172-2297 / +55 21 3172-1896

Cover design: Thieme Publishing Group
Typesetting by DiTech Process Solutions

Printed in the United States of America by King Printing
                                  5 4 3 2 1

ISBN 978-1-62623-806-0

Also available as an e-book:
eISBN 978-1-62623-807-7

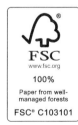

FSC
www.fsc.org
100%
Paper from well-
managed forests
FSC® C103101

Contents

Preface   viii

Introduction   ix

1   Symptom-Focused Care of the PDLS   1

2   Fundamental Anatomy   4

3   Spinopelvic Parameters and Sagittal Balance   22

4   Stabilization in SFC Surgery on the PDLS   31

5   Clinical Evaluation of the Patient with a PDLS   40

6   The Fundamental Open Surgical Method   57

7   Lateral Intramuscular Planar Approach for
     Instrumentation/Stabilization L3 to Sacrum   87

8   Minimally Invasive Surgical Method   93
     James B. Macon

9   Postoperative Care   122

10   Surgical Situations of Complex Decision-Making   129

11   Socioeconomics in Spine Surgery   137

Index   147

Preface

"Is there anything so wise as to learn by the experience of others?"

—Voltaire

For the last 3 years, after 31 years in private practice, I have had the great pleasure of being a member of an academic neurosurgery program. The Carilion Neurosurgery Department has afforded me the opportunity to focus on degenerative spine surgery, which is, and has been for some time, the area of my primary interest.

I had no idea that working with diligent, stimulating, and enthusiastic residents could be so enjoyable. But I have also learned that their considerable responsibilities in a busy general neurosurgical practice, at a Level I trauma center, affords them little time (either in the clinic or the OR) to develop the fundamental clinical and technical skills necessary for the care of patients with degenerative spine pain.

The learning curve in the care of the painful degenerative lumbar spine is a long one. This is partly because the pathology in any given patient has a singular character. The anatomy of that pathology always varies in some degree, so that it will not be precisely alike any other. Furthermore, the multi-variant clinical factors in any patient can never be the exact same as in any other patient. The experienced surgeon therefore should have significant instructive value, clinically and operatively, to the young surgeon willing to learn what is still, to a large degree, an art.

This book is not primarily meant to be a technical treatise. For instance, it is not so concerned with the specifics of the technique in the various types of lumbar fusion. It is more concerned, however, with identifying the patient who needs a fusion, and why a particular fusion method for that individual patient is the best option.

And yet as degenerative lumbar spine surgery mainly concerns itself with various techniques of neural decompression, the principles of these methods will be presented, some of which may not be generally understood and practiced. The *en-bloc laminectomy* technique, for example, has been developed as a safe and effective technique for the most severe cases of lumbar stenosis. Similarly, there is the description in the use of bony landmarks for navigating a challenging decompression on a multi-operated spine. The far-lateral *LIMP Approach* to the lower lumbar spine and sacrum[1] its technical refinement and applications have not been presented outside its original presentation.

This book will provide a thorough overview of the fundamental clinical knowledge and evaluative techniques needed to make the best therapeutic decision for each individual patient. And as with the technical aspects, there will be presentation here of novel clinical concepts. Specifically, in the evaluation of chronic low back pain, a *descriptive clinical sub-classification system* is suggested. And in patients with chronic (mechanical) axial low back pain, *a grading scale* is presented based on a simple testing maneuver. This scale has been of considerable value to me in surgical decision-making for this group of patients, as will be discussed.

These techniques and evaluative methods have been honed over 35 years of neurosurgical practice which has included an extensive and intensive experience with degenerative spine disease. And yet I remain on the learning curve, though hopefully leveled out somewhat. It is my wish that this experience will be used to enhance the advancement of young spinal surgeons along this clinical curve.

The proper surgical care in the patient with the painful degenerative lumbar spine (PDLS) is not clarified in many areas. I have added an "Unknowns and Investigational Opportunities" section, when appropriate, to emphasize those areas needing further study. As symptom-focused care is *individualized care*, and as individual clinical factors are interactively complex, there will never be the establishment of immutable algorithms in the surgical care of the painful degenerative lumbar spine (PDLS). But we can continue to increase our knowledge on *pathophysiologic processes.*

The development of this increasing knowledge base is associated with, and affected by, the socioeconomic environment. It is my opinion that changes in this environment in recent years have been, in many ways, deleterious to honest and valid scientific investigation, and thus to clinical direction. I have therefore closed this text with a final chapter on socioeconomics. A strong case could be made that this chapter is the most important contribution for the young spinal surgeon, because the consequences of the present socioeconomic climate, if unchanged, will ultimately deprive him/her of the freedom of ethical care for their patients.

Reference

1. Weaver EN. Lateral intramuscular planar approach to the lumbar spine and sacrum. *Journal of Neurosurgery: Spine.* 2007;7 (2):270–273. doi:10.3171/spi-07/08/270.

Introduction

The current surgical literature on the painful degenerative lumbar spine (PDLS) is replete with technical articles, often informing as to nuances and modifications of some form of spinal stabilization. But there has been a relative dearth of information pertinent to the processes of surgical evaluative decision-making. As spinal surgeons, we have become quite adept at various techniques in the OR and are ever-improving these abilities and their requisite tools; many patients have benefitted accordingly. But in recent years, the published investigational science of these technical developments has been excessively dominant at the expense of the clinical science dealing with the appropriate application of these newer techniques and tools. This dominance can be attributed, in no small degree, to economic influences—some quite subtle and indirect, others more overt (see Chapter 11, "Socioeconomics in Spinal Surgery").

There is no sub-specialty in medical science where acumen in the clinical evaluation of the individual patient has more import. This pertains to the fact that a patient's symptomatology is mainly subjective. *The fact that surgery on the degenerative spine is primarily pain surgery cannot be over-emphasized.* In the great majority of patients, the pain of operative consideration is *radicular* though surgery for non-radicular pain may also be indicated in selected cases of true axial mechanical pain.

Our patients are very complex entities. He or she is a human organism with an abstruse emotional and cognitive substratum underlying a subjective pain complaint. We often must factor in multiple personal and social issues, as well as the anatomical/physiologic ones, before deciding on the best therapeutic approach for any given patient; in so doing, we are continuing in the practice of surgery on the painful degenerative lumbar spine as "an art."

The Current Stress on Ethical Professionalism

The advent of spinal instrumentation has changed the mindset of the spinal surgeon away from that advocated by Dr. Osler. Today, he might introduce another sentence to the above quote in reference to the surgical treatment of the PDLS: "The mediocre physician treats the radiograph."

Surely the tools of instrumentation have given the degenerative spine surgeon mechanisms for safer and better treatment of certain pathologies which require stabilization (fusion). But this "hardware" in its multitudinous forms, and with hundreds of ancillary and niche products, *is expensive, and thus profit-making.* Spinal fusion in the patient with PDLS has become an international multi-billion dollar industry.

The current ethical stress on the profession of spinal surgery is, in main part, the consequence of the fact that spinal surgeons have been incorporated into the profit stream of this industry. Our financial involvement has taken many forms, the most pernicious of which occurs when we are involved in establishing the clinical validity of a product in which we have personal financial interest. In this COI scenario, published instrumentation research is unavoidably corrupted (see Chapter 11, "Socioeconomics in Spinal Surgery").

Not only has the economic influence of this industry clouded our investigation into clinical validity of instrumentation, but we are also ethically challenged in their use by a healthcare policy of "intervention-based" reimbursement. Payment for our surgical services is done based on the number of interventions (each represented by a special code number) per surgical procedure, and these interventions are weighted as to difficulty/magnitude. The use of instrumentation not only adds another interventional charge, but a large one at that.

Fundamentally, instrumentation is used for the correction or stabilization of radiographic deformity. Hence in trauma or in major deformity/

scoliosis surgery, its use is *primarily* determined by radiographic evaluation, and surgical decision-making is usually straightforward. However, in spinal surgery on the PDLS, any such correction/stabilization is *secondary* to the primary intent of pain relief. In these cases, the indications for instrumentation are less defined, and their clarification needs ongoing valid investigation.

It is this area, surgery on the PDLS, wherein is our greatest ethical challenge. The economic dynamics have resulted in our fixation on instrumentation. We find our mindsets have shifted from the primary goal of patient pain relief, in the most limited manner possible, to one of viewing radiographs and defining appropriate therapy as instrumented deformity correction. This shift from a primary diagnostic emphasis on the pain symptomatology to that of radiographic abnormality has been subtle yet trenchant.

To many of us, especially our younger colleagues, the therapeutic significance of symptom-focused evaluation is often wanting. These young surgeons may not be exposed to a process of an intense and personal clinical evaluation. Many are untrained in the communicative ability to probe and identify the true cause of the patient's suffering, which may or may not be primarily pain. Thus they may render a surgical plan based primarily on radiographic presentation, in the absence of a vigorous query of the specifics of symptomatology. They may not appreciate the significance, for instance, that almost every patient suffering from primary depression also has an "abnormal" MRI.

And yet, mostly, they are highly intelligent, diligent, responsible, and caring. They simply have not been *taught* a more symptom-focused care approach to the care of these patients.

1 Symptom-Focused Care of the Painful Degenerative Lumbar Spine (PDLS)

Abstract

Symptom-focused care of the painful degenerative lumbar spine defines a clinical philosophy whereby the surgeon, by intensive interaction with the patient, establishes precisely the patient's primary complaint. With rare exception, such complaint is described as some form of pain. The surgeon must then determine the etiology of the presenting pain complaint and thus establish, at least tentatively, a **diagnosis**. It is necessary for the surgeon to have the expertise to identify non-surgical and/or non-spinal etiologies, and it is incumbent on him/her, as physicians first and surgeons second, to address some therapeutic approach for non-surgical pathologies.

SFC surgery for the PDLS is primarily focused on relief of the presenting pain, requiring, in most instances, some form of root decompression. The decision for surgery is primarily a **clinical** one and is **individualized,** respective of the innumerable pertinent factors variable from patient to patient. Image evaluation, usually MRI, is used to confirm radicular compression at the site congruent with that determined by clinical evaluation.

In SFC surgery of the PDLS, fusion/instrumentation is mainly done adjunctively as a prophylactic measure, avoiding the potential for increasing instability. Image-defined spinal deformity, therefore, is not a primary imperative and its correction is relevant only to adequate root decompression. This absence of any compulsion for deformity correction is, relatively, surgery-limiting and can be considered a **minimalism** surgery. This clinical minimalistic approach is differentiated from mini-invasive surgery (MIS) which is a technical term. Minimalism surgery defines "what" surgery is to be done; MIS describes methodologically "how" the surgeon may accomplish it.

Keywords: diagnosis, individualized, minimalism, mini-invasive, MIS, deformity

As to diseases, make a habit of two things— to help, or at least, to do no harm. To do nothing is sometimes a good remedy.

Hippocrates

1.1 The Professional Obligation in the Examining Room

Symptom-focused care (SFC) is an approach to the patient with PDLS, which is fundamentally established through an extensive personal interaction between the patient and the surgeon. Emphasis is placed on delineating precisely and specifically the patient's primary complaint. The emphasis on SFC may seem to be unnecessary to some who would imagine, and expect, that all surgeons treating the PDLS would approach their patients accordingly. Unfortunately, in recent years, there have been subtle but cogent forces that have resulted in a clinical shift rendering the emphasis on symptom-based care secondary to that based on image pathology.

In a large majority of potential surgical cases with incapacitating degenerative spine symptomatology, the primary complaint involves some description of pain. This suffering of pain will often include a socioemotional component requiring an attentive and compassionate evaluative history. It is our covenantal obligation, as physicians/surgeons, to attempt elucidation of all such factors in the patient's pain complaint. In so doing, we may find that an emotive component is a predominant factor. The identification of significant situational social duress and/or depression is critical to therapeutic decision-making.

With SFC, the surgeon's imperative is to establish a diagnosis. This conclusion may be tentative, requiring further investigation; but with attention to the whole patient, it must have some initial definition. The SFC surgeon is firstly a *physician* attempting to relieve *suffering*, whatever the cause(s). Often, a surgical option will not be the appropriate choice after further elucidation of all factors defining the patient's suffering.

The patient has not come to serve the surgeon, but rather the reverse. **There should be little professional ethical tolerance for the surgeon who evaluates the patient solely in terms of the decision as to whether or not that patient is a surgical candidate**. The fact that many patients have a form of suffering for which surgery is not the remedy does not absolve the surgeon from establishing a diagnosis and directing appropriate therapy. The surgeon must be knowledgeable and competent in the clinical evaluation of various nonradicular causes of pain presentation, including any of socio-psychogenic relevance. If the surgeon is not so informed, then significant nonspinal pathology will be missed. Moreover, inappropriate surgery will be done when surgical blinders direct a fixation only on spinal etiologies, disregarding other possibilities.

The physical examination in the patient with degenerative spine pain is essential. Yet, it is less informative for diagnostic and/ or therapeutic direction than is face-to-face verbal communication with the patient. The exam may reveal neurologic (root) compromise and thus confirm suspected localization gained from the history; but only rarely is the examination the sole directive of surgical therapy unassociated with a pertinent and consistent history of pain.

Image evaluation (mainly magnetic resonance imaging [MRI]) in SFC secondarily confirms the tentative diagnosis established clinically, with a consistent conformation of a structural compressive mechanism. MRI "abnormalities" are ubiquitous in the degenerative spine, and the surgeon must establish congruency between the presenting pain complaint and any image abnormality. Without clear MRI confirmation of a compressive pathology at the clinically appropriate site, the surgeon must consider other etiologies or otherwise account for the discrepancy.

Spinopelvic and global alignment. In SFC surgery on the PDLS, stabilization procedures are secondary and limited (see Chapter 4: "Stabilization in SFC Surgery on the PDLS"). Any deformity correction is only consequent to such needed stabilization. However, there is growing evidence that, even in short-segment stabilization (1–3 levels), balance parameters should be assessed especially in regard to the development of junctional stress. Furthermore, the SFC surgeon will be assigned to treat patients who may need more aggressive global deformity procedures. Hence, the SFC surgeon must have thorough knowledge of regional and global balance parameters, and their application; these will be discussed extensively in subsequent chapters.

1.2 SFC Surgery on the PDLS Is Primarily Decompressive

Operative techniques in SFC surgery are standard, depending on the surgeon's preference. However, in certain difficult and complicated surgical cases, decompressive techniques require an expertise not readily gained in the practice of image-directed spinal surgery (trauma and deformity surgery).

Thus, SFC surgery is based on a thorough clinical evaluation supported by appropriate image pathology. Its focus is specifically on the segmental structural abnormality causing the patient's symptoms. As such, **SFC surgery is minimalist surgery**, although with prophylactic considerations when appropriate. Accordingly, deformity and/or balance parameters may have such relevance.

Minimally invasive surgery (MIS) is applicable to SFC surgery (see Chapter 8: "Minimally Invasive Surgical Method). MIS is a *technical term*, referring to a procedural method to accomplish a defined operative goal. SFC surgery refers to a *clinically based minimalist directive* that establishes the most limited surgical intervention to remedy the individual patient's symptomatology. Yet, this limited focus must be considerate of the long-term effects, especially as it relates to underlying pathophysiology.

1.3 Stabilization in SFC Surgery on the PDLS Is Mainly Adjunctive

The use of pedicle screw (PS) instrumentation, mainly in support of bony arthrodesis, has become commonplace in the surgical treatment of the PDLS, especially when image studies show evidence of potential translational "instability" represented by spondylolisthesis. There has been the concern that a definitive decompression at that level will predispose for further vertebral displacement. Investigation into defining the clinical and radiographic factors for the risk of this progression, in relation to various decompression techniques, has been relatively sparse until recently; hence, fusion/instrumentation techniques have been done on a routine basis when the radicular pain pathology involves operation at a level of radiographic spondylolisthesis. Current literature suggests that many of these slips are stable and that prophylactic instrumentation is not necessary when limited decompression techniques are used (see Chapter 10: "Surgical Situations of Complex Decision-Making").

The addition of interbody cages may add to the stability of a PS construct by adding anterior strut support and increasing potential for bony arthrodesis. In addition to their effect on stability, these techniques may contribute directly to decompression with expansion of the vertebral interspace and subsequent opening of the foramina. The advent of expandable cages has enhanced this capability and has also given the surgeon an additional technique for limited sagittal correction.

As noted, stability procedures in degenerative SFC surgery are usually planned secondarily as a necessary adjunct to the primary goal of appropriate root decompression for amelioration of pain. *However, in cases of incapacitating mechanical (antigravity) chronic axial lumbar pain (CALPag), stabilization may be definitively therapeutic.* Such CALPag may be addressed as the patient's sole dysfunctional pain syndrome, or it may exist as a significant component with radicular pain, as is seen sometimes with recurrent lumbar disc herniation. Only an SFC approach to the patient will make the proper determination as to the need for stabilization in either of these scenarios.

2 Fundamental Anatomy

Abstract

A spatial understanding of the skeletal anatomy is crucial for the surgeon. Bony landmarks are used for guidance to neural compressive pathology. In the degenerative and/or pre-operated spine, normal anatomic features are distorted, imbedded in cicatrix, or absent. Safe root decompression in such circumstances can be challenging and the surgeon often must do so by dissecting along the "lateral corridor" which is the inter-connecting pathway of the facet joints, the pars interarticularis, and the inferior articular processes. The dynamic anatomy of the dorsal vertebral connections is complex. In normal anatomy, each facet joint has a stabilization contribution from the contralateral side. There are five ways by which the surgical removal of bone can destabilize a facet. The particular architecture of the joint also has relevance to this stability.

The classical depiction of muscle anatomy (and their differentiating planes) at the lower lumbar region is erroneous. A better understanding of this anatomy will allow the surgeon to use the lateral intramuscular plane for dissection to the lateral vertebral/pedicle region. Functionally, the lumbar musculature can be divided into three main groups: multifidus, pars thoracis, and pars lumborum. These groups are arranged for spinal stability during elevational movement of the spine much like cables supporting the boom of a construction crane.

For the surgeon, important knowledge of the neural anatomy is primary in reference to the nerve roots. The dermatomal distributions of their ventral rami, especially, allow for more specific delineation of the pain generating compressive process. Anatomical variation of root anatomy must also be understood especially as it pertains to conjoined nerve roots which can be damaged if their presence is unappreciate after review of the MRI, or at surgery. The afferent nociceptive neural pathways from the skeletal and discogenic spine are not clearly understood and there is evidence that sympathetic innervation/pathways may be involved. The gate control theory of somatic pain transmission accounts for clinical features of pain and also for the paradoxical pain of root compression.

Keywords: lumbar musculature, lumbar skeletal, facet joint, facet destabilization, transitional vertebrae, lumbo-sacral plexus, dermatomes, gate control theory, sympathetic nerves, sinovertebral

Get the fundamentals down and the level of everything you do will rise.

Michael Jordan

Reference Note:

Much of the following anatomic presentation is drawn from *Clinical Anatomy of the Lumbar Spine and Sacrum*, 4th ed., by Bogduk and Endres.[1] The reader is directed to this invaluable text as a companion reference for clarification and review. Additional illustrations here are provided when they have particular clinical/operative relevance.

2.1 Space Definitions

- Subarticular space: below medial edges of facets through which root travels prior to entering foramen (► Fig. 2.1).
- Lateral recess: same as "subarticular space."
- Foramen: space extending laterally under pars and limited superiorly (cephalad) and inferiorly (caudally) by pedicles.

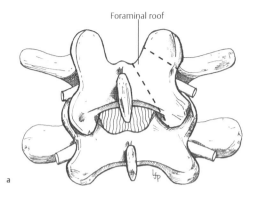

Foraminal roof

Fig. 2.1 **(a)** Foraminal roof: dorsal margin of foramen. **(b)** Lateral margin of foramen.

a

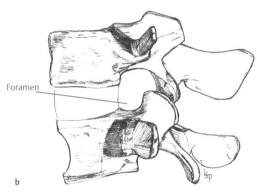

Foramen

b

- Foraminal or intraforaminal: within space of foramen.
- Intracanalicular: all space in canal medial to foramen.
- Extraforaminal: space lateral to foramen (edge of pars).
- Safe sublaminar space: The epidural space below the superior lateral half of each lamina is between the attachments of the ligament flava to that lamina. It is dorsal to the lateral aspect of the dural sac and approaches the medial aspect of the exiting root. Thus, it provides the surgeon with a relatively safe space for exposure/passage without jeopardy to the dura and nerve root (▶ Fig. 2.2).

2.2 Muscular Anatomy

The classic depiction of the lumbar musculature, as divided by vertical sagittal planes,[2] is not wholly accurate at the lowest lumbar levels.[3] For the surgeon, it can be simplified into three *functional* components at the lower lumbar levels.

- The ***multifidus*** is the largest component. It consists of overlapping bundles of paraspinous fibers that remain medial to the lateral edge of the facets (encompassed by a shiny fascia) extending caudally to the L4–L5 joint. Importantly, at this level, the fibers fan out to the ilium/sacrum with the most lateral part extending nearly horizontally into the ilium. Thus, these fanning fibers roof the more caudal lumbosacral articulation.

The multifidus, primarily oriented along the spinous processes, provides functional dynamic stability of the vertebrae in relation to each other. At its caudal end, it is anchored at the ilium/sacrum, and the ilial

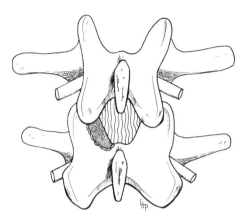

Fig. 2.2 Relatively safe access to epidural space under lamina between attachments of ligamentum flavum.

attachment is robust and nearly transversely oriented. The medial fibers of the multifidus are vertically oriented, attaching at right angles to the posterior margins of the spinous processes. This orientation establishes the multifidus' vector of action as primarily that of posterior sagittal rotation (and resistance to anterior rotation). This vector allows for relatively minimal resistance to anterior translation.

- The **pars thoracis** of the erector spinae musculature (longissimus thoracis and iliocostalis lumborum) is represented by the aponeurosis of erector spinae (AES) extending from the level of L3 caudally, merging with the fascia of the multifidus medially, and constituting the deep fascia at these lower levels. There may be some pars thoracis muscle fibers medially (i.e., on the underside of the AES adjacent to the lateral fascia of the multifidus).

The primary function of the pars thoracis is related to its connection from the pelvis to the thorax, mainly spanning the lumbar region, and is involved in stabilization of the upper body in response to gravitational forces. Thus, it allows for a controlled gravitational descent in bending, and for tension stabilization and lifting in the action of elevating the upper body in relation to the pelvis. The action of pars thoracis in the upright position increases lumbar lordosis (posterior rotation) and its unilateral action produces lateral flexion.

- **Pars lumborum** of the erector spinae has also been classically separated into components of the longissimus thoracis and the iliocostalis lumborum. However, the function of these two components is essentially similar. Together, they attach at each level from the ancillary and transverse processes, inserting on the lateral ilium and an aponeurotic cephalad extension from this (lumbar intermuscular aponeurosis). Their main vector of action is horizontal (posterior), adding antitranslational resistance. Their vertical vector can produce lateral coronal and posterior rotational force.

Construction crane analogy: The human, as an upright biped, must have the capacity to interact physically with the ground and so must have the capacity to re-erect to an ambulatory status from that level. Evolutionary forces have created an efficient muscular/mechanical system to this effect. Certain types of construction cranes have been engineered with a stabilization system analogous to the human anatomic one (▶ Fig. 2.3).

- **Lateral intramuscular plane:** a distinct fatty plane of separation exists between the pars lumborum and the multifidus below L3. This plane is directed to the

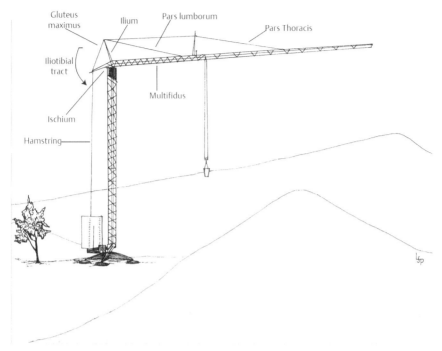

Fig. 2.3 Construction crane demonstrating correlation of its lifting and stability mechanics with that of the human anatomy.

juncture of the transverse process and superior articular process. In contradiction to the usual anatomical depiction, this plain is not vertically sagittal; rather, it is oblique. At its upper portion (L3–L4), this obliquity is longitudinal with the axis of the spine. At L5–S1, this obliquity turns laterally toward the ilium, thus following the lateral edge of the multifidus in a **J**-shaped curve. This plane can be found just medial to the ilium and provides a clear avenue of access for stabilization procedures at these levels (▶ Fig. 2.4).

2.3 Skeletal Anatomy

A thorough and three-dimensional understanding of the anatomy of the lumbar vertebral bodies and sacrum/ilium, and their interconnections, is essential. The bony anatomy here represents the signposts directing to the neural elements needing

decompression. Certain landmarks are crucial for appropriate instrumentation application. These anatomic features will be represented in the technical presentations of this book.

2.3.1 Operative Landmarks to the Lateral Corridor

In certain instances, the normal anatomy has been distorted either through degenerative changes or from previous surgery(s). In the latter situation, technical difficulties arise from previous bony removal and/or from obscurity rendered by cicatrix. Thus, the surgeon must often identify a bony landmark and use it as a road map to advance to the pathology needing decompression via *the lateral corridor*. There are two such main landmarks and their directive relationship to the roots must be understood:

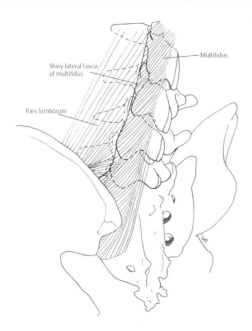

Fig. 2.4 Lateral intramuscular plane as oblique and "**J**" shaped.

Shiny lateral fascia of multifidus

Multifidus

Pars lumborum

1. The spinous process/lamina: If this is present, it can be followed down/laterally to safely access the appropriate root:
   - Inferiorly (caudally) along the medial inferior articular process (IAP) for access to the root that is enumerated one greater than the designated number of the associated spinous process.
   - Superiorly (cranially) along the pars to access the root of same enumeration as the spinous process (▶ Fig. 2.5).

Both of these approaches lead to the facet joint, which is the other major landmark and which can be used to advance decompression sequentially further caudally and/or cephalad.

2. The facet joint: Often, the spinous processes have previously been removed and a facet joint can be found safely by dissection laterally. The medial aspect of the joint will direct the surgeon to the underlying root either to its proximal portion by exploring along the IAP or more distally at the foramen by exploration at the pars. Importantly, once the joint is exposed, the surgeon can advance caudally along this *lateral corridor* from pars–lamina–IAP to next facet, etc. (or cranially: IAP–lamina–pars to facet, etc.), for multiple root decompressions with less danger of dural disruption than in attempts to establish root anatomy from a more medial position (see Chapter 7) (▶ Fig. 2.6).

2.3.2 Zygapophyseal (Facet) Joints

Functional integrity: The surgeon must know the functional stabilization/destabilization anatomy of the facet joints, with the understanding that the stability of a facet joint has contribution *from the contralateral side*. This knowledge is important in the consideration of various techniques for root decompression. *Five ways in which facet destabilization* can occur are:

1. The loss of functional integrity of the superior articular process/facet (rare).
2. The loss of functional integrity of the IAP/facet (▶ Fig. 2.7).

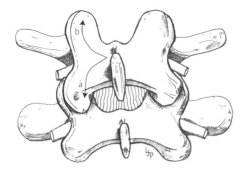

Fig. 2.5 Access to lateral corridor by following intact spinous process to lamina.

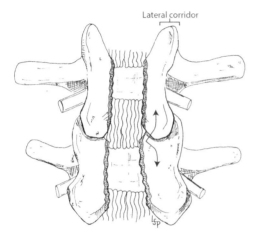

Fig. 2.6 Access to lateral corridor by direct exposure of intact facet.

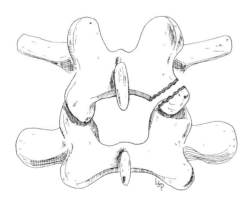

Fig. 2.7 Facet destabilization from loss of structural integrity of inferior articular process.

3. The loss of functional integrity of both struts of the IAP—the ipsilateral pars and the ipsilateral lamina (▶ Fig. 2.8).
4. The loss of functional integrity of the ipsilateral pars and the contralateral lamina (▶ Fig. 2.9).
5. The loss of functional integrity of both pars (bilateral facet joint destabilization) (▶ Fig. 2.10).

It should be understood that with the rare exception of #1 above, the instability induced involves the defective vertebra and the next caudal one. Thus, in the common case of stenosis at a level of degenerative (nonisthmic) spondylolisthesis at L4–L5, a unilateral far distal decompression of the symptomatic L5 root will be across the L5 pars and thus have no effect on stability of L4–L5 slip (▶ Fig. 2.11).

Architecture

• There are two pertinent features of facet architecture: the shape of the articulating surfaces and their orientation in regard to the sagittal plane. The articulating surfaces can be cupped into a "**C**" or "**J**" shape or can be relatively flat. The sagittal orientation can range from near 0 degrees (vertical = superior facet facing opposite side) to near 90 degrees (horizontal = superior facet facing posteriorly).

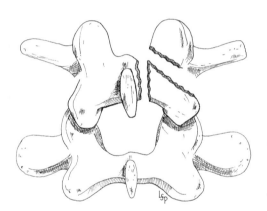

Fig. 2.8 Facet destabilization by loss of structural integrity of the two struts of the IAP: ipsilateral lamina and pars.

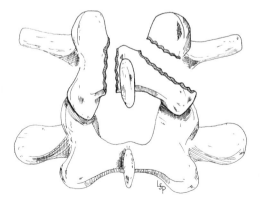

Fig. 2.9 Facet destabilization from loss of structural integrity of ipsilateral pars and contralateral lamina representing bilateral contribution to stability.

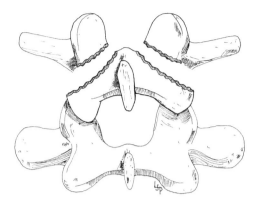

Fig. 2.10 Bilateral facet destabilization from loss of structural integrity of both pars.

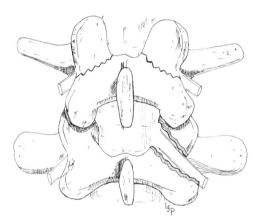

Fig. 2.11 Unilateral parsectomy, with laminal intact, does not destabilize the facet.

- In regard to stability: the more horizontal the superior facet, the greater the resistance provided to translational displacement of the upper vertebra (anterolisthesis). Vertical joints have greater potential for anterolisthesis but allow for sagittal rotation. Normally, the facet orientation is more vertical in the higher lumbar levels to accommodate sagittal rotation in bending. At the lower levels, the orientation becomes more horizontal in order to resist the significant gravitational translational forces exerted in the upright position.
- At any orientation, cupped/J-shaped facets have greater resistance to displacement than flat facets.

- The L4–L5 and L5–S1 joint sagittal orientations generally range from 30 to 75 degrees; however, a small percent at either level may have a significantly greater vertical orientation subjective to anterior displacement forces (i.e., development of spondylolisthesis).
- Above L4–L5, the normal orientation is progressively more vertical (accommodating rotation).

Joint Capsule

- The fibrous capsule of the facet joint is most robust in the dorsal aspect.
- At the superior and inferior poles, the capsule is redundant with adipose

tissue filling the resulting subcapsular pocket. This fat communicates with the extracapsular space through a small foramen.

- Anteromedially, the fibrous capsule is replaced by the ligamentum flavum attachment to the facet margin. *The removal of this attachment, with exposure of the anterior/medial joint space, does not result in any appreciable weakening of the joint.*

2.3.3 Ligaments

Ligamentum flavum: From a surgeon's technical perspective, the anatomy of the *ligamentum flavum* has the greatest relevance. Accordingly, several points will be emphasized:

- This is a paired (bilateral) symmetric ligament connecting successive vertebrae. Attachment to the upper vertebra is to the pedicle and the inferior third/half of lamina and the medial IAP. This extends caudally and divides into two distinct parts or leafs. The *ventral part (leaf)* continues to the lower vertebra attaching to the superior/ventral aspect of its lamina. A *superficial leaf* attachment is to the medial edge of the facet joint (forming its anterior capsule) and to the dorsal aspect of the lower vertebral lamina/pars. This

leaf can be removed with preservation of the ventral leaf still attached to the lamina (▶ Fig. 2.12). This superficial leaf attachment to the facet is of minimal structural significance to joint stability and can be removed surgically without consequence.

- Medially, the ligament is continuous, forming the ventral third of the ipsilateral interspinous ligament angling dorsocranially.
- The thinner ventral leaf attachment to the superior lamina of the vertebra below is to its upper edge and ventral surface. *The thinness and superficiality of this ligamentous attachment allows for safe entry into the epidural space especially at L5–S1.*
- Once the superficial leaf to the facet is removed, and the ventral leaf is detached from the lamina, the *safe sublaminar space* (see Space Definitions, above) can be developed laterally under the lamina to the proximal foramen/pedicle area. *This allows for a relatively safe approach to the nerve root at the foraminal entrance, which is lateral/distal to common pathology within the vertebral canal* (▶ Fig. 2.13).

Iliolumbar ligament: This is a multilayered ligamentous complex extending from the lateral body of L5 and its transverse process

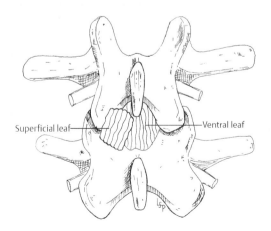

Fig. 2.12 Two leaves of ligamentum flavum: superficial (attachment to medial facet) and deep (between laminae).

Superficial leaf —— Ventral leaf

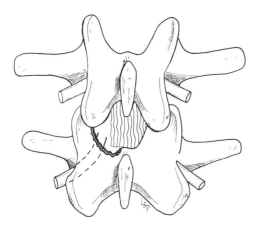

Fig. 2.13 Root identification following development of safe sublaminar space laterally.

to the ilium. It is a strong attachment that prevents forward displacement at the lumbosacral junction (anterolisthesis of L5).

- Anteriorly, the upper aspect of this ligament forms the attachment of the quadratus lumborum muscle.
- At its lower aspect anteriorly, the ligament has vertical fibers, which form the lateral aspect of the channel through which the L5 ventral ramus enters the pelvis.

The development of this ligament is felt to proceed from muscular tissue in children to a nearly full ligamentous state by the third decade. *Conceptually, an abridged progress of this development may be a factor in the subsequent occurrence of isthmic spondylolisthesis. And, conversely, an accentuated osteoblastic development could account for transitional variants.*

2.3.4 Lumbosacral Transitional Vertebrae (as per Castellvi)

- **Castellvi** radiographic classification system (TPL5 = transverse process of L5):
  - Type I: enlarged (> 19 mm height) TPL5: unilaterally (IA) or bilaterally (IB).

- Type II: TPL5—sacral *articulation*: unilaterally (IIA) or bilaterally (IIB).
  - Type III: TPL5—sacral *fusion*: unilaterally (IIIA) or bilaterally (IIIB).
  - Type IV: any bilateral *combination* of above pathology[4] (▶ Fig. 2.14).
- Transitional vertebra have been related to radiographic degenerative change and to lumbar curvature (lordosis).[5]
- The evidence for a relationship between transitional vertebrae and "chronic low back pain" is controversial. The prevalence of transitional vertebrae in the asymptomatic population may not be significantly different (lower) from that in the patients with back pain.[6]

Sacroiliac Joint

- The function of the SI joints is to relieve stress from forces (transmitted through the pelvis) between the upper body and the lower extremities.
- Thus, the SI joint is designed to withstand longitudinal (gravitational) stress as well as torsional stresses applied from ambulatory movement of the legs.
- The ranges of motion of the SI joint are very small (1–2 degrees)—mainly in posterior rotation.

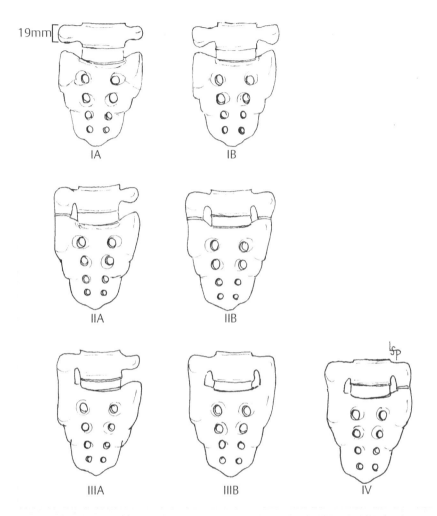

Fig. 2.14 Castellvi classification showing progression from increased TP height of L5 (IA,B) to articulation (IIA,B) to fusion (IIIA,B).

- Motion restraint is established by the interlocking bony contour of the surfaces and by abundant ligamentous connection anteriorly (sacroiliac ligaments) and posteriorly (interosseous and posterior sacroiliac ligaments).
- The lower sacrum also has ligamentous support to the ischium (from below the SI joint), thus providing further anterior rotational restrain to the sacrum.

- Innervation of the SI joint has not been well established, but the best evidence suggests that it includes posterior and ventral rami contribution from L3 to S3. *This multisegmental innervation may have relevance to the protean presentation of clinical pain description in patients with purported SI joint pathology.*

2.4 Neurological Anatomy

2.4.1 Somatic Nerves

- Nerve **rootlets** are divisions[1,3-5,7-13] of nerve **roots** connecting to the spinal cord; **ventral** (mainly motor) **rootlets** attaching to the ventrolateral aspect and **dorsal** (sensory) **rootlets** attaching to the dorsolateral sulcus.
- A segmental **ventral root** and **dorsal root** extend intrathecally (each encased within pia mater) from rootlets and converge into a dural sleeve (sheath) at each level; they continue to the termination of this sleeve within the intervertebral foramen and merge to form the short **spinal nerve** (the extension of the dura of the sleeve becomes the epineurium of this spinal nerve).
- Immediately proximal to this merger of the roots, the dorsal root forms into the **dorsal root ganglion**, which comprises the cell bodies of the sensory fibers. This ganglion is a visible enlargement of the distal dural sleeve at the upper and medial region of the intervertebral foramen.

- At the exit of the foramen, the spinal nerve divides into a **ventral ramus** and **dorsal ramus**.
- The dorsal ramus divides into a lateral, intermediate, and medial **branch** at all levels except L5 (which has no lateral branch).
- The combined ventral rami form (within the psoas muscle) either the **lumbar plexus** (L1–L4) or the **sacral plexus** (S1–S3). The former coalesces into peripheral nerves that (with the exception of the obturator nerve) run anterior/superior to the pelvic rim (e.g., femoral nerve); the latter forms nerves that traverse posterior/inferior to the pelvic rim (e.g., sciatic nerve) (▶ Fig. 2.15).
- The L5 ventral ramus (with a branch from L4) forms the **lumbosacral trunk** which connects the two plexuses, the entirety sometimes referred to as the **lumbosacral plexus**. *It is important to note that the lumbosacral trunk must pass anterior to the sacral ala to merge with the sacral elements. Thus, it angles diagonally, dorsal to ventral, across the lateral L4 intervertebral disc.*

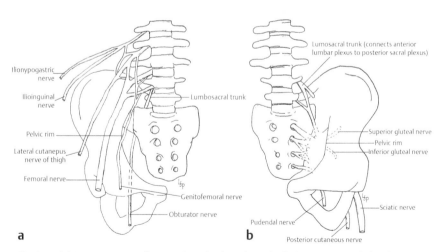

Fig. 2.15 **(a)** Representation of nerves from lumbar plexus (with the exception of the obturator nerve) emerging anterior to pelvic rim. **(b)** Representation of nerves from sacral plexus emerging posterior to pelvic rim. The lumbosacral trunk is connecting the two plexuses by angling dorsal/posterior to ventral/anterior in line with the lateral margins of the L4 and L5 intervertebral discs.

2.4.2 Conjoined Nerve Roots

- Various classification schemes describe anomalous nerve root anatomy.
- The conjoined nerve root (CNR) is one such anomaly whereby two pairs (dorsal and ventral) of roots exit the dural sac through a common root sleeve.
- The CNR has particular morphologic relevance to surgery: it is significantly larger than a normal root, and its aberrant position in the foramen can be at the level of the disc.
- The CNR is not inherently symptomatic, although its size and position can effect painful symptomatology with relatively minor degenerative pathology (i.e., small herniated nucleus pulposus [HNP] and/or minimal stenosis) and thus patients may present symptomatically without compelling compressive pathology radiographically. However, most symptomatic CNRs occur with disc herniations that are radiographically overt.
- Clinically, the symptomatic CNR presents with back pain/radicular symptoms with or without clinical clues: bidermatomal representation or dermatomal distribution inconsistent with level of HNP pathology.
- The magnetic resonance imaging (MRI) scan may provide asymmetric signs strongly suggestive of the CNR with or without evidence of disc herniation.[8]
  - "Sagittal shoulder sign": on sagittal views, a vertical space-occupying structure connecting the exiting root with (apparent) traversing root behind a herniated disc (may represent large exiting CNR at level of disc).
  - Asymmetric presentation in T1 axials of extradural fat in the spinal canal at foraminal level:
    a) Small crescent-shaped fat between dural sac and CNR ("fat crescent sign").
    b) Truncated dural sac within the fat ("corner sign").
  - Asymmetric root presentation on T1 axials:
    a) Obvious asymmetrically enlarged root sleeve.
    b) Absence of foraminal root (suggestive of conjoined root at adjacent level).
    c) Two root images visualized in same foramen ("axial common passage sign").
    d) Visualization of entire course of root at disc level (due to its horizontal disposition and often associated with "corner sign").
- The T2 coronal MRI and the myelogram/computed tomography (CT) (water-soluble contrast) are most useful tools in evaluating and/or confirming presence of CNR.

2.4.3 Sympathetic Nerves (and Their Interconnection with Somatic Nerves)

- The anterior spinal column is surrounded by an interconnecting neural plexus (**circumferential plexus**). It is subdefined into the **anterior**, **lateral**, and **posterior plexuses**. This circumferential plexus has direct somatic contribution from the ventral rami and direct sympathetic contribution from the sympathetic trunks and gray rami communicantes (GRCs).
- The **sympathetic trunks** extend along the anterolateral vertebral column adjacent to medial edge of psoas major muscle. Each trunk has, on average, four ganglia. They have multiple interconnections in the space anterior to the vertebral bodies/discs in the **anterior plexus**.
- One to three **GRCs** extend from the sympathetic trunk to each lumbar ventral rami, passing through tunnels posterior to the psoas muscle and connecting with the ventral rami just outside the intervertebral foramen. Only the ventral rami of L1 and L2 also receive **white rami communicantes** (**WRCs**).
- The **GRCs** also contribute to the lateral part of the circumferential plexus

(**lateral plexus**) and make an autonomic contribution to the **sinuvertebral nerves (SVNs)**.

- The **SVNs** are recurrent branches from each ventral ramus which enter into the canal and parallel the lateral edge of the posterior longitudinal ligament, ascending from the disc/ligament of entry to the next higher disc/ligament. These nerves also contribute to the nerve plexus along the floor of the canal (**posterior plexus**). The SVNs are mixed nerves having both a somatic component/root from ventral rami and the sympathetic contribution/root from the **GRCs** (▶ Fig. 2.16).

2.4.4 Innervation

Spinal Musculature

- The multifidus (and interspinous) muscles are supplied by the medial branch of the dorsal ramus. *Importantly,* the medial branch adheres to a strict segmental distribution: it innervates only

those muscles that arise from the lamina and spinous process of the vertebra, which is numbered the same as the spinal nerve of its origin.

- The longissimus is supplied by the intermediate branches of the dorsal rami.
- The iliocostalis lumborum is supplied by lateral branches of the dorsal rami.

Skin (via Dorsal Rami)

- Only the lateral branches of the dorsal rami become cutaneous.
- The skin of the lumbar area is innervated by the dorsal rami of L1, L2, and L3.
- The lateral branch of L1 most commonly becomes cutaneous to supply the skin of the buttocks from the lateral iliac crest (7–8 cm from midline) to the greater trochanter. Contributions may exist from L2 and L3 (via superior cluneal nerve).
- Cutaneous contribution from the L4 lateral branch is uncommon.
- There is no consistent dorsal ramus cutaneous contribution from L5, as it has no lateral branch.

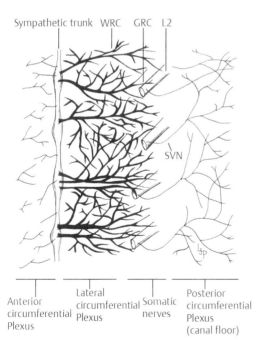

Sympathetic trunk   WRC   GRC   L2

SVN

Lsp

Anterior circumferential Plexus

Lateral circumferential Plexus

Somatic nerves

Posterior circumferential Plexus (canal floor)

Fig. 2.16 Schematic representation of interconnections between the circumferential plexus, the sympathetic trunk, and the somatic nerves.

Skin (via Ventral Rami = Dermatomal)

- Each spinal nerve and its dorsal root receive sensory fibers, via ventral ramus, from a defined dermatomal distribution.
- The lumbar dermatomal distributions are variable and overlapping but each spinal nerve has an autonomous dermatomal zone, which is relatively (but not completely) consistent in different individuals (▸ Fig. 2.17).

Intervertebral Discs

- The lumbar discs and adjacent ligament are supplied by the posterior plexus with SVN contribution from same level and the adjacent lower level.
- Somatic afferent fibers from these structures may return to the ventral ramus via the SVNs or via circumferential plexus.

- There is evidence that there is a sympathetic afferent pain pathway from the intervertebral discs entering centrally via the L2 spinal nerves. Presumably, this pathway involves the SVNs to the lateral plexus and/or sympathetic trunk and then via the WRCs to the L2 nerve. Thus, discogenic back pain, via this pathway, would be considered analogous to visceral pain.[9,10]

2.4.5 Pain Pathways

Ascending

- Pain pathways are highly complex with other secondary tracts and polysynaptic projections.
- Receptor = nociceptor: stimulated by tissue damage. (Note: receptors may be predominantly free nerve endings; transduction of impulse to fibers is not well understood.)

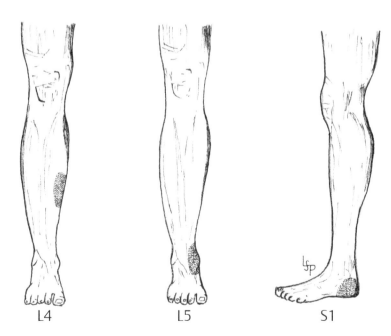

Fig. 2.17 Relative autonomous dermatomal zones.

- Nociceptors: have high threshold to natural stimuli and can be *sensitized* (progressively augmenting response to repeated or increasingly noxious stimuli).
- Transmission to spinal cord dorsal horn by two types of *small* fibers: A-delta fibers and C fibers
- A-delta fibers are myelinated and provide rapid transmission (at 17 m/s) of impulse.
- C fibers are unmyelinated and transmit considerably more slowly (at 1 m/s).
- Central transmission is done mainly via dorsal root ganglion/dorsal roots but *recurrent fibers from dorsal root ganglion may enter ventral root* (perhaps 15–30% axons in ventral roots are sensory).
- At the dorsal horn, these fibers excite projection neurons mainly in the marginal layer (lamina I) but also in lamina V (of nucleus proprius), and also synapse with interneurons at levels of the substantia gelatinosa (laminae II, III).
- The projection neuron transmits the second-order nociceptive afferents via the contralateral medial and lateral spinothalamic tracts to the thalamus, mainly to the ventroposterolateral and posterior nuclei. (There are multiple collateral projections of the spinothalamic tracts: medial reticular formation, periaqueductal gray, nucleus cuneiformis, and sub- and hypothalamus).
- Substance P is probably a primary afferent transmitter for noxious stimuli.

Descending Control of Pain

- Electrical stimulation of the periaqueductal gray and brainstem reticular formation, and especially the raphe nuclei, produces analgesia by suppressing spinal unit activity (naloxone reversible).
- Pathways mainly involve dorsolateral fasciculus (tract of Lissauer) but also via ventral and ventrolateral funiculi.
- Cortical and pyramidal stimulation has been shown to suppress the activity of spinothalamic neurons by unknown mechanisms.

2.4.6 The Gate Control Theory of Pain (of Melzack and Wall) [11,14]

- Interneurons (probably in substantia gelatinosa) exhibit a *tonic* suppressive effect on the second-order projection neuron.
- C-fiber nociceptive impulses exert suppressive effect on the interneuron (as well as excitatory to the projection neuron), potentiating its excitation and hence "opening the gate" for pain transmission (▶ Fig. 2.18a).
- *Large* myelinated and rapid-transit (30–60 m/s) fibers from mechanoreceptors/touch receptors likewise have an excitatory effect on the projection neuron. However, they also excite the interneuron, which results in increased suppression of the projection neuron, thus "closing the gate" for pain transmission (▶ Fig. 2.18b).
- Descending modulatory control systems are also factorial in the Melzack and Wall theory.
- The gate control theory accounts for the phenomena of some pain relief by rubbing of a painful area. Similarly, it is the basis for therapeutic electrical transcutaneous stimulation (i.e., TENS).
- *The gate control theory also accounts for the paradoxical pain response to nerve root compression (e.g., by a herniated nucleus pulposis): the large nonnociceptive myelinated fibers are more susceptible to mechanical compression than the smaller nociceptive fibers and thus their increased relative dysfunction will remove excitatory stimulus to the suppressive interneuron and thus "open the gate" for pain transmission* (▶ Fig. 2.18c).

2.5 Unknowns and Investigational Opportunities

- Clear delineation of lumbar muscular anatomy with emphasis on intermuscular plane configuration.

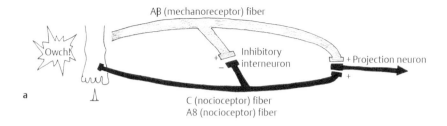

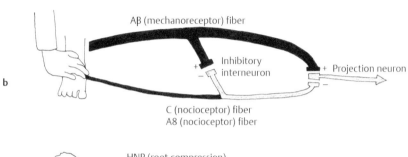

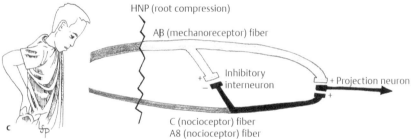

Fig. 2.18 (a) Opening the gate: by nociceptive fiber stimulation which suppresses the tonic inhibition of the interneuron and excites the projection neuron. **(b)** Closing the gate: by large rapid-transit fibers from mechanoreceptor /touch receptor stimulation which increases excitation of tonic inhibitory interneuron. **(c)** Paradoxical response of pain with nerve/root compression which opens the gate by preferentially blocking large rapid-transit fiber impulses removing excitation stimulus to inhibitory interneuron.

- Establishment of muscular/mechanical mechanism(s) of re-erection from the standing flexed position.
- Innervation and afferent nociceptive pathway from annulus fibrosis (i.e., "discogenic" axial lumbar pain): level of centralization; role of sympathetic plexus.
- Innervation and afferent nociceptive pathway for skeletal pain: role of

sympathetic plexus; role of intraosseous (perivascular) sympathetics.

References

[1] Bogduk N, Endres SM. Clinical Anatomy of the Lumbar Spine and Sacrum. London: Churchill Livingstone; 2005
[2] Palmer DK, Allen JL, Williams PA, et al. Multilevel magnetic resonance imaging analysis of

multifidus-longissimus cleavage planes in the lumbar spine and potential clinical applications to Wiltse's paraspinal approach. Spine. 2011; 36(16):1263–1267

[3] Weaver EN, Jr. Lateral intramuscular planar approach to the lumbar spine and sacrum. Technical note. J Neurosurg Spine. 2007; 7(2):270–273

[4] Castellvi AE, Goldstein LA, Chan DP. Lumbosacral transitional vertebrae and their relationship with lumbar extradural defects. Spine. 1984; 9(5): 493–495

[5] Mahato NK. Disc spaces, vertebral dimensions, and angle values at the lumbar region: a radioanatomical perspective in spines with L5-S1 transitions: clinical article. J Neurosurg Spine. 2011; 15 (4):371–379

[6] Apazidis A, Ricart PA, Diefenbach CM, Spivak JM. The prevalence of transitional vertebrae in the lumbar spine. Spine J. 2011; 11(9):858–862

[7] McCulloch JA, Waddell G. Variation of the lumbosacral myotomes with bony segmental anomalies. J Bone Joint Surg Br. 1980; 62-B(4):475–480

[8] Trimba R, Spivak JM, Bendo JA. Conjoined nerve roots of the lumbar spine. Spine J. 2012; 12 (6):515–524

[9] Ohtori S, Nakamura S, Koshi T, et al. Effectiveness of L2 spinal nerve infiltration for selective discogenic low back pain patients. J Orthop Sci. 2010; 15(6):731–736

[10] Nakamura SI, Takahashi K, Takahashi Y, Yamagata M, Moriya H. The afferent pathways of discogenic low-back pain. Evaluation of L2 spinal nerve infiltration. J Bone Joint Surg Br. 1996; 78(4):606–612

[11] Melzack R, Wall PD. Pain mechanisms: a new theory. J Pain. 1996; 5(1):3–11

[12] Murata Y, Takahashi K, Yamagata M, Takahashi Y, Shimada Y, Moriya H. Sensory innervation of the sacroiliac joint in rats. Spine. 2000; 25(16): 2015–2019

[13] Smucker JD, Akhavan S, Furey C. Understanding bony safety zones in the posterior iliac crest: an anatomic study from the Hamann-Todd collection. Spine. 2010; 35(7):725–729

[14] Moayedi M, Davis KD. Theories of pain: from specificity to gate control. J Neurophysiol. 2013; 109 (1):5–12

3 Spinopelvic Parameters and Sagittal Balance

Abstract

Preoperative attention to sagittal alignment is a clinical necessity in the longer stability constructs of degenerative deformity/scoliosis surgery. For shorter constructs in SFC surgery on the PDLS, the kinematics of junctional stress may provide less of an imperative for aggressive sagittal correction. Though adjacent segment disease (ASD) is a realistic concern in these cases, more precise indications for sagittal correction have not yet been established. And individual variances of other pertinent clinical factors may not allow a logrhythmic approach to care for this group of patients. But the degree of sagittal misalignment is an important factor in the over-all individual equation defining the need for, and extent of, sagittal correction.

Sagittal alignment parameters are skeletal measurements, taken in the standing position, usually describing some relationship between the spine and the pelvis. As true global alignment is in reference to whole-body balance around the feet (i.e. Dubousset's "cone of economy") these spinopelvic parameters have some limitation in defining direct gravitational stress on the lumbar spine.

The most common spinopelvic measurements are based in plumb-line variance. The sagittal vertical axis (SVA) for instance measures the distance between the plumb-line (vertical) from the centroid of C7 and the posterior/superior corner of S1. The accuracy of plumb-line measurements will be distorted when compensatory mechanisms are used to achieve a better balance of the upper body over the pelvis; the rotation of the hip on the femoral axis and knee-bending are the main such mechanisms. Other non-plumb-line spinopelvic parameters may be independent of such compensation. These may accurately reflect gravitational stress of the upper body on the lumbar spine and thus useful

to the PDLS surgeon. The measured reciprocal difference between the pelvic incidence and lumbar lordosis (PI-LL) is commonly used to calculate sagittal correction needs. The T1 pelvic angle is another such parameter which obviates the need for compensatory measurement (e.g., pelvic tilt) when deciding on the need for surgical sagittal correction.

Keywords: cone of economy, gravity line, spinopelvic parameters, pelvic incidence, pelvic tilt, sacral slant, sagittal balance, sagittal vertical axis, T1pelvic angle, lumbar lordosis

Get knowledge of the spine, for this is the requisite for many diseases.

Hippocrates

3.1 Introduction

In major scoliosis surgery, recent data have demonstrated the significance of sagittal misalignment in lumbar pain/disability as well as a causative factor in kinematic and degenerative changes of the lumbar spine.[1,2,3] In the more limited and segmental PDLS surgery of symptom-focused care (SFC), sagittal balance evaluation may have relevance to surgical planning in certain scenarios. These pertain to cases where a short-segment *stabilization procedure may be indicated as integral to symptomatic therapy* and the potential/degree of postoperative junctional stress is assessed. There is evidence that the development of adjacent segment disease in short-segment stabilization has a strong correlation with *regional* spinopelvic imbalance.[4] Thus, evaluation of sagittal parameters in these instances may influence the *extent* of sagittal correction needed, and thus the techniques adjusted accordingly. There is also evidence that sagittal imbalance may have relevance to the outcome of multisegment decompression for stenosis.[5] (These considerations will be examined in more detail in Chapter 4.)

Specific indications of sagittal balance evaluation and correction, in these instances, need further elucidation. Furthermore, patient-specific modifiers will influence the surgeon's evaluation as to the relevance of these considerations. However, it is important that the PDLS surgeon understands these metrics as, assuredly, they will be factorial in the surgical decision-making as relevant to outcome in certain patients.

3.1.1 Spinopelvic Parameters

The bony pelvis is a unified structure (minimal sacroiliac joint movement) and functions as the platform foundation on which the spine is based. Its rotary function on the femoral head is essential for use of hands at the ground level, for sitting, for re-erection to the upright position, and for bipedal ambulation. The pelvic structure has individual morphologic variation. Such variation has effect on the standing spinopelvic relationship (as well as with locomotion). Specifically, during growth/development, the platform morphology of the pelvis will have formative influence on the spine's ultimate shape, as it responds to the constant force of gravity in maintaining a balanced position.[6,7] As overall (global) balance is established to the feet, through the rotational fulcrum at the hips, the relationship between the pelvic platform and the femoral heads also has influence on the morphologic development of the spinal structure.

- The **pelvic incidence (PI)** represents the fixed inclination of the axis of the sacrum relative to the pelvic acetabula. In adults, it is a morphological parameter inherent to each individual. It is measured as the angle formed by the line from the midfemoral axis (bicoxofemoral axis)

to the center of the sacral end plate and the other line from this point perpendicular to the end plate. Thus, the greater this angle, the more inclined the sacral axis is relative to the overall pelvis, as represented by a greater slope of the sacral end plate (▶ Fig. 3.1). The slope of the S1 end plate may vary (slightly) from the perpendicular of the sacral axis, also having effect on the measured PI; a third factor in determining the PI, inherent to any given patient, is the location of the S1 end plate along the sacral axis. Thus, if the sacral end plate is higher and more anterior, the PI will be represented as a smaller angle, and the reverse if it is lower/posterior. With normal segmental anatomy, this end plate variation is negligible. However, in the situation of a transitional level with complete or partial sacralization of L5 (four lumbar vertebrae) or lumbarization of S1 (six lumbar vertebrae), the level of the end plate can create a significant variation in measured PI (▶ Fig. 3.2).

- **Lumbar lordosis (LL)** is a relatively fixed parameter measured as the Cobb angle from the superior end plate of T12 (or L1) to that of S1. The relationship

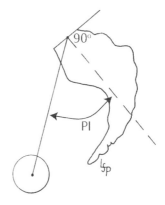

Fig. 3.1 Pelvic incidence (PI): a fixed individual angle describing inclination of sacral axis within skeletal pelvis.

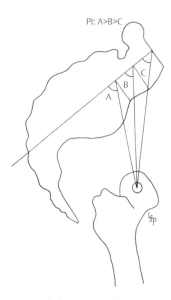

PI: A>B>C

Fig. 3.2 PI is variable individually dependent on level of sacral end plate.

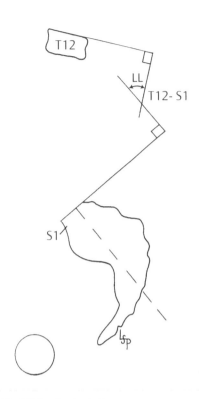

T12

LL

T12- S1

S1

Fig. 3.3 Lumbar lordosis.

between the PI and the LL will establish a segmental sagittal alignment from T12 to the acetabula. The PI and the LL would be close to equal to establish T12 neutrally above the acetabula (normal variance, ± 10 degrees). It should be noted that, normally, the LL is predicted by the PI. At low PI (30–40 degrees = flatter sacral end plate), the normal curve at the L4 and L5 motion segments provides adequate lordosis, with either a neutral or a kyphotic upper lumbar curve. As the PI increases, the higher lumbar motion segments are progressively recruited, with the consequence of moving the apex of the lordotic curve cranially. In effect, the L1 and L2 motion segments crucially fine-tune the LL according to the PI. The understanding of this relationship may have consequence in segmental reconstruction[8] (▶ Fig. 3.3).

- The **sacral slant (SS)** refers to the angle formed by the sacral end plate and the horizontal. It is unfixed in that it varies as to any rotation of the pelvis over the femoral heads (▶ Fig. 3.4).

- The **pelvic tilt (PT)** measures the rotation of the pelvis at the hip. Thus, anterior rotation is the primary mechanism of movement in bending forward. However, posterior rotation (retroversion) has a much more limited range. It is represented by a hip extension. The PT measures this rotation as the angle formed by the anterior PI line (femoral heads to central sacral end plate) and a vertical plumb line. Hence, as the pelvis rotates anteriorly, this PI line will rotate similarly relative to the fixed plumb line and the PT will become smaller in degree (and becomes a negative value when it passes the plumb line). In retroversion, PT becomes larger. The SS necessarily varies inversely with PT in pelvic rotation: with anterior rotation (PT decreasing), the sacral end plate inclines more vertically (relative to the horizontal) and thus SS increases. In retroversion, this angle lessens as PT increases (▶ Fig. 3.5).

- **PI = SS + PT:** As PI is a fixed value for any individual, the inverse relationship between PT and SS establishes this

equation. Thus, a major compensatory mechanism (PT) is established as the measureable difference between PI and SS (PI − SS = PT). An elevated PT (either directly measured or calculated) is a sign of sagittal imbalance compensation by pelvic restoration.

3.1.2 Global Balance and Compensatory Mechanisms

Center of Mass and Gravity Line

Dubousset described the "cone of economy," which is defined "by the range of sway of the center of mass relative to the feet that can be readily accommodated by the structural elements and musculature of the standing individual."[1] Importantly, the cone of economy refers to the overall balance in reference to the feet. In normally balanced individuals, force-plate evaluation establishes that this cone revolves around a gravity line (GL) extending from the feet (at the level of the anterior tibia cortex) through the femoral heads, and with a constant offset to T9.[9] The position of the center of mass in any individual is a function of spinal morphology and of soft-tissue

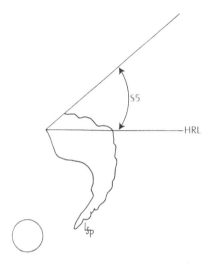

Fig. 3.4 Sacral slant (SS): variable with pelvic rotation.

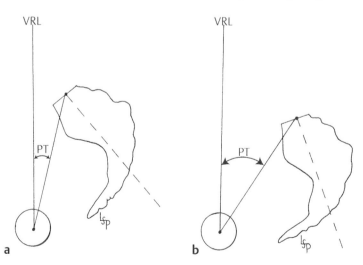

Fig. 3.5 **(a)** Pelvic tilt (PT): the measure of rotation. **(b)** Pelvic tilt (PT): increases in retroversion inversely and proportionately with SS.

25

distribution. With abnormal balance, the soft-tissue mass is a static component, and the patient (and surgeon) can effect corrective maneuvers for imbalance only by skeletal manipulation. The direction of an abnormal global balance can exist toward any place on the cone's circumference depending on the summation of lateral (coronal) and anterior-posterior (sagittal) balance.

In adult spinal deformity surgery (with long stabilization constructs), sagittal alignment has strong correlation with outcomes,[10] whereas coronal deformity has less operative consequence.[10] With sagittal imbalance, the individual's center of mass is either anterior or posterior to the "economic" position, resulting in a GL deviation from its normal position relative to anatomic landmarks: in positive sagittal imbalance, it would angle (from the feet) anterior to its usual anatomic course, and in negative sagittal balance, it would angle posterior to it.

In the present context, abnormal sagittal balance is consequent to spinal degenerative deformity. Underlying inherent morphologic variation of the pelvis may affect this aging dynamic process. The disposition of soft tissue, in extreme cases of obesity, may be an independent factor in affecting the center of mass and balance, and thus degenerative deformation. Although there is minimal information in regard to obesity and sagittal balance, obesity has been established as an independent factor in the development of multisegmental spondylosis.[11]

Compensatory Mechanisms

When an individual is imbalanced in the sagittal plane, in the upright position he/she will attempt to achieve a compensatory standing posture that maximizes muscular economy (and thus physical comfort). This will entail mechanisms to move the center of mass back to a more normal GL relative to the feet. Those in negative sagittal balance have an ample range of flexion at the hip, which is a relatively efficient compensatory mechanism, accomplished by rotating

the pelvis anteriorly on the femoral heads. However, hip extension compensation for positive sagittal imbalance is more problematic, as the resulting minimal anterior translation, with its posterior rotation (retroversion), has a limited range (± 10 degrees). If further movement of the center of mass posteriorly is necessary, then the knees and ankles will be flexed. This will tilt and translate the pelvis further backward.[9]

The evaluation of compensation for positive sagittal balance would entail measurement of:

- Pelvic retroversion (posterior rotation of pelvis on femoral heads): PT greater than normal.
- Knee-flexion angle.
- Posterior pelvic translation: pelvic shift (▶ Fig. 3.6).

3.1.3 Evaluation of Sagittal Balance

Spinal radiographs are used to assess global sagittal balance and its compensation; although without a capability of establishing the center of mass, there are limitations to the correlation of these measures with full-body sagittal balance assessment as determined by force-plate evaluation. Most of these parameters are based on a plumb-line relationship between the spine and the pelvis, whereas true global balance is referenced to the feet. Thus, changes of hip and lower extremity joint position can affect the accuracy of spinopelvic radiographic measurement of global balance.

Sagittal Measurement Based on Plumb-Lining

- The **sagittal vertical axis (SVA)** is the most common measurement of sagittal balance. It is a measurement of the sagittal deviance of the plumb line from the centroid of C7 to the posterior/superior corner of S1. Positive and negative values reflect anterior and posterior deviance, respectively. In general, a positive value

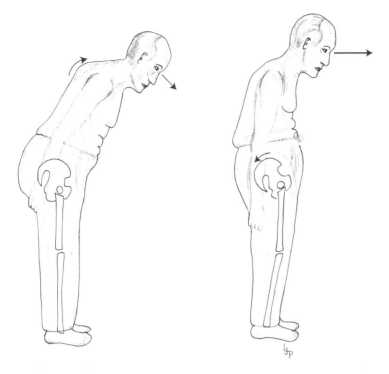

Fig. 3.6 Postural compensation for sagittal imbalance: pelvic retroversion and knee flexion (without forced reduction of lordosis).

of < 50 mm is considered normal and a value of > 80 mm is considered severe imbalance (▶ Fig. 3.7). However, normal sagittal balance is variable with age. (See "rules of thumb" below.)

The accuracy of this measurement alone in the assessment of global sagittal balance can be severely limited by any rotation at the hips. An individual who is compensating for negative balance with such flexion may be incorrectly determined as balance-neutral. Or an individual with unrecognized flexion-contracture at the hip can be deemed severely positively imbalanced.

- Other spinopelvic plumb-line measures of global balance include the **T1 spino-pelvic inclination** and the **T9 spinopel-vic inclination**.[10] These measure the angle formed by the line from the respective vertebral body to the femoral

head (or bicoxofemoral axis) with the plumb-line (vertical) through that same femoral point. As measured relative to the plumb, they will vary with hip rotation and so their accuracy is dependent on this and other compensation maneuvers.
- The plumb-line from the **cranial center of mass** may be an important and reliable marker of global spinal balance.[12]

Sagittal Balance as Fixed Angular Measurements of the Spine in Relation to the Pelvis

The plumb-line measurements address the relationship between some point of the upper body spine and a fixed point on the pelvis. Plumb-line variance is measured as a distance or as an angle. As noted earlier, this measurement can be affected by

27

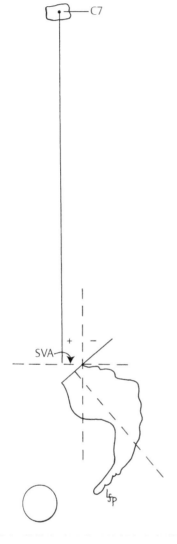

Fig. 3.7 Sagittal vertical axis: measured positive or negative in reference to posterior corner of sacral end plate.

rotation and/or translation of the pelvis by compensatory mechanisms. Other indicators of the sagittal relationship between the spine and the pelvis can be measured as a fixed angular function, irrespective of gravitational effect (i.e., plumb-line). These measurements are therefore not affected by

compensatory positioning of the pelvis. But it must be emphasized that these too represent regional skeletal alignment parameters and are not direct measures of global alignment (i.e., deviance from gravity line).

Relationship between Pelvic Incidence and Lumbar Lordosis (PI–LL)

The PI is an individual inherent pelvic parameter that measures the inclination of the S1 end plate with regard to the axis of hip rotation (acetabula; ▸ Fig. 3.2). Thus, it measures morphologic variation of the pelvic platform to which the axial vertebral spine is attached (see below). The steeper the slant of this platform, the greater the PI measurement. The vertebral spine must be adjusted to this slant in order to position the body within the efficient "cone of economy": this entails a lordotic position of L1 essentially above the acetabula. Therefore, the greater the inclination of this platform (SS), the more lordosis of the lumbar spine needed to accomplish this position. The measured SS in the standing position can vary with rotation of the pelvis; the PI, however, is the measurement of the platform that is fixed to the axis of hip rotation and thus is invariable by pelvic movement. Thus, the PI–LL is a parameter with relatively minimal variation in any individual patient. It is considered normal at < 10 degrees. And as this measurement does not account for the curvature of the thoracic/cervical spines, it is not a singular measure of global sagittal balance. However, it can be considered a primary parameter, which influences the development of the more cephalad thoracic and cervical curves in response to gravitational force. It may have particular relevance to short-segment stabilization on the PDLS.[4]

- **Sagittal tilt (ST)** refers to the angle formed by a line from the C7 centroid to the center of the sacral plate and the anterior horizontal. Any angle less than 90 degrees indicates the center of C7 is anterior to the sacral plate. Normal positive and negative range of this angle is approximately 7 degrees.[10]

- The **T1 pelvic angle (TPA)**[13,14,15,16] is another proposed spinopelvic parameter that is not plumb-line based. It accounts for sagittal misalignment in an easily measured angle formed by the line from the femoral head axis to the centroid of T1 and the line from that axis to the middle of S1 end plate (normal is < 15 degrees and severe deformity is > 20 degrees; ▶ Fig. 3.8). This parameter appears to have promise for PDLS surgeons in the assessment of preoperative sagittal misalignment; it is an intrinsic measurement independent of rotational compensatory mechanisms of the pelvis (pelvic retroversion or forward flexion at the hips). However, it is dependent on both the lumbar and thoracic curvatures. As such, it may have a value in preoperative planning in SFC surgery on the PDLS when short-segment stabilization is needed and in patients with neurogenic claudication secondary to lumbar stenosis in regard to the potential for outcome degradation secondary to persistent/progressive back pain.

Sagittal Vertical Axis and TPA Versus Patient Age (Numbers Adopted and Rounded Off from Lafage et al[17])

- Age < 45: SVA (mm) decreasingly negative approaching neutral; TPA (degrees) < 10.
- Age 45–55: SVA and TPA increasing to 15.
- Age 55–65: SVA increasing to 35; TPA increasing to 20.
- Age 65–75: SVA increasing to 55; TPA increasing to 25.
- Age > 75: SVA increasing to 75; TPA increasing to 30.

Rule of thumb ("15 /55 + 20 /10"): Until the age of 55 years, both SVA (mm) and

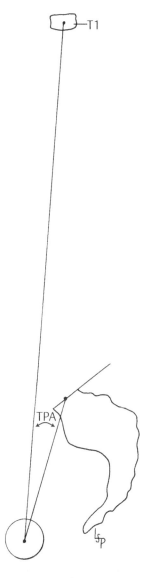

Fig. 3.8 T1 pelvic angle (TPA): sagittal relationship of upper thoracic spine with sacrum, without reference to plumb-line variable only by spine curvature.

TPA (degrees) are less than 15. For each decade following, add 20 mm (2 mm/year) to the SVA and 5 degrees (0.25/year) to the TPA.

- **Surgical implication:** In the younger patients who undergo PDLS stabilization surgery, restoration to normal age-related sagittal parameters may prevent progressive deformity with aging, the use of age-averaged parameters could result in under-correction in younger patients.

3.1.4 Coronal Plane Metrics

The imperative of sagittal balance evaluation in adult degenerative scoliosis surgery is established based on outcome measures.[10] There is early and compelling evidence that, in the short-segment stabilization of PDLS surgery, regional sagittal evaluation (PI–LL) may be important for optimal results.[4]

In stabilization surgery by the PDLS surgeon, global coronal alignment evaluation is necessary in the frequent setting of lumbar degenerative scoliosis. The interrelationship between any pelvic obliquity, scoliosis, and possible leg-length discrepancy must be determined (see Chapter 4).

Global coronal alignment: It is assessed as the horizontal distance from the C7 plumb-line to the center of the sacrum. A neutral coronal alignment is 0, and misalignments to the left and right are, respectively, designated as negative and positive. Deviance of > 4 cm is considered abnormal.

Pelvic obliquity: It is noted visually on the standing lumbar anterior-posterior radiographs. It is commonly measured as an angle with the horizontal reference using the line along the ilia. Other pelvic landmarks can be used.[10]

Leg-length discrepancy: In cases of pelvic obliquity (tilt) noted on standard X-rays, anterior-posterior standing radiographs, to include lumbar spine and feet (with knees locked), are necessary to allow for accurate leg-length measurement.

References

[1] Ames CP, Smith JS, Scheer JK, et al. Impact of spinopelvic alignment on decision making in deformity surgery in adults: a review. J Neurosurg Spine. 2012; 16(6):547–564

[2] Vrtovec T, Janssen MMA, Likar B, Castelein RM, Viergever MA, Pernuš F. A review of methods for evaluating the quantitative parameters of sagittal pelvic alignment. Spine J. 2012; 12(5):433–446

[3] Keorochana G, Taghavi CE, Lee K-B, et al. Effect of sagittal alignment on kinematic changes and degree of disc degeneration in the lumbar spine: an analysis using positional MRI. Spine. 2011; 36(11):893–898

[4] Rothenfluh DA, Mueller DA, Rothenfluh E, Min K. Pelvic incidence-lumbar lordosis mismatch predisposes to adjacent segment disease after lumbar spinal fusion. Eur Spine J. 2015; 24(6):1251–1258

[5] Graham RB, Sugrue PA, Koski TR. Adult degenerative scoliosis. Clin Spine Surg. 2016; 29(3):95–107

[6] Funao H, Tsuji T, Hosogane N, et al. Comparative study of spinopelvic sagittal alignment between patients with and without degenerative spondylolisthesis. Eur Spine J. 2012; 21(11):2181–2187

[7] Lee J-H, Kim K-T, Suk K-S, et al. Analysis of spinopelvic parameters in lumbar degenerative kyphosis: correlation with spinal stenosis and spondylolisthesis. Spine. 2010; 35(24):E1386–E1391

[8] Anwar HA, Butler JS, Yarashi T, Rajakulendran K, Molloy S. Segmental Pelvic Correlation (SPeC): a novel approach to understanding sagittal plane spinal alignment. Spine J. 2015; 15(12):2518–2523

[9] Ferrero E, Liabaud B, Challier V, et al. Role of pelvic translation and lower-extremity compensation to maintain gravity line position in spinal deformity. J Neurosurg Spine. 2016; 24(3):436–446

[10] Annis P, Brodke D. Lumbar region. In: Haid R, Schwab F, Shaffrey C, Youssef J, eds. Global Spinal Alignment Principles, Pathologies and Procedures. 1st ed. St. Louis, MO: Quality Medical Publishing; 2015:165–188

[11] McCormick P. Lumbar spine disease: considerations for obese patients. AANS Bulletin. 2008; 17(2)

[12] Sugrue PA, McClendon J, Jr, Smith TR, et al. Redefining global spinal balance: normative values of cranial center of mass from a prospective cohort of asymptomatic individuals. Spine. 2013; 38(6):484–489

[13] Ryan DJ, Protopsaltis TS, Ames CP, et al. International Spine Study Group. T1 pelvic angle (TPA) effectively evaluates sagittal deformity and assesses radiographical surgical outcomes longitudinally. Spine. 2014; 39(15):1203–1210

[14] Qiao J, Zhu F, Xu L, et al. T1 pelvic angle: a new predictor for postoperative sagittal balance and clinical outcomes in adult scoliosis. Spine. 2014; 39(25):2103–2107

[15] Protopsaltis T, Schwab F, Bronsard N, et al. International Spine Study Group. The T1 pelvic angle, a novel radiographic measure of global sagittal deformity, accounts for both spinal inclination and pelvic tilt and correlates with health-related

quality of life. J Bone Joint Surg Am. 2014; 96 (19):1631–1640

[16] Diebo BG, Ferrero E, Lafage R, et al. Recruitment of compensatory mechanisms in sagittal spinal malalignment is age and regional deformity dependent: a full-standing axis analysis of key radiographical parameters. Spine. 2015; 40 (9):642–649

[17] Lafage R, Schwab F, Challier V, et al. International Spine Study Group. Defining Spino-pelvic alignment thresholds. Spine. 2016; 41(1):62–68

4 Stabilization in SFC Surgery on the PDLS

Abstract

Stabilization in SFC surgery on the PDLS is mainly done adjunctively to address translational instability or rotational hypermobility at the level of planned root decompression. It may also be done as a primary therapeutic maneuver in mechanical (antigravity) chronic axial lumbar pain (CALPag). It is also indicated in most cases of symptomatic adjacent segment disease (ASD) after a previous fusion.

The relationship between sagittal imbalance (SIB) and ASD, in short-segment fusion, has not been completely elucidated, though lordotic enhancement techniques should be considered in any patient with SIB needing arthrodesis. In rare cases when stabilization is planned, but with severe SIB, aggressive lumbar lordotic correction may require osteotomy(s).

Root decompression at a mid-lumbar level with significant coronal deformity may require stabilization to prevent progressive cephalad deformity. Also, when stenotic root decompression is needed at the convexity of a coronal curve, stabilization with some deformity correction may prevent recurrence.

In the setting of coronal lumbar scoliosis, an evaluation for leg-length discrepancy is an imperative. If a coronal curve is convex secondarily to an ipsilateral shorter leg, then the post op stability and clinical effectiveness of correction will be in jeopardy.

Keywords: index disc degeneration, junctional kyphosis, adjacent segment disease, sagittal imbalance, coronal deformity, pelvic obliquity

We must however acknowledge, as it seems to me, that man with all his noble qualities … still bears in his bodily frame the indelible stamp of his lowly origin.

Charles Darwin

4.1 Introduction

Presently, the term "stabilization" infers the establishment of a bony arthrodesis (fusion) in the great majority of cases done today. However, nonfusion stabilization techniques exist, and newer ones are being developed, mainly in an attempt to limit the junctional stress issues (discussed later). It is anticipated that there will be further development of these "dynamic" or "motion preservation" stabilization techniques, and that their use will become increasingly more common.[1]

4.2 The Dynamic Component in the Progression of Degeneration/Deformity from Index Disc Degeneration: The Role of Gravitational Force

The extent and form in the development of lumbar degenerative changes is a complex interactive function between inherent anatomic/physiologic features and subsequent physical stresses. Common pertinent anatomic features include variances in the lumbosacral transition (i.e., transitional vertebrae), shape and position of the sacral platform (i.e., affecting pelvic incidence [PI]), and leg-length discrepancy. Physical factors are the common and unavoidable antigravity stresses rendered to the bipedal upright human, and which are variant depending on body habitus/mass. These anatomic and physical factors impact on inherent metabolic variances in the disposition for degenerative disc change and bone density, which in turn can be affected by behavioral influence (diet, smoking, drug/medications, environmental toxins).

The resultant degenerative disc disease of the lumbar spine occurs within an upright individual who must move vertically back and forth from the ground (lying, sitting, bending, squatting) to the upright position. In these antigravity motions, muscular forces act on the vertebral elements, and this muscle action is necessarily asymmetric.

Importantly, degeneration/deformity at an index level can lead to reactive degeneration/deformity at other level(s). As there is use of the natural flexibility leverage of the thoracic spine to compensate for any resulting imbalance, secondary degenerative/deformity forces are exerted in segments adjacent to an index level. Thus, a biomechanical change at one lumbar level can affect adjacent levels, creating a domino effect on overall degeneration/deformity of the spine: "Multiple spondylitic and arthropathic segments contribute to a vicious pathogenic cycle, leading to dynamic biomechanical shifts, such as spondylolisthesis and rotatory subluxation, throughout the lumbar spine, and thus a degenerative deformity occurs."[2]

The understanding of these dynamics may be important for the PDLS surgeon in order to plan any limited stabilization surgery. The PDLS surgeon must be facile with various balance and spinopelvic parameter measures in order to incorporate them into operative planning. Sagittal balance, particularly, has relevance to outcomes,[3] although its accurate measurement can be problematic and must take into account compensatory mechanisms (see Chapter 3).

Presently, there is limited investigational evidence relating operative outcomes of short-segment stabilization to preoperative sagittal evaluation. The evaluation of this relationship would necessarily focus on the biomechanical stresses on the transitional area and the clinical consequences thereof. One well-designed retrospective study has shown a strong correlation between adjacent segment disease (ASD)

and PI–lumbar lordosis (PI–LL) mismatch of > 10 degrees.[4] A greater specificity of those patients needing sagittal correction will be established by further investigation as to the concomitant role of global and/or regional imbalance and the size/position of the stabilization construct.

4.3 The Issue of Postoperative Junctional Stress: Adjacent Segment Disease and Junctional Kyphosis

The rigidity of the spine incorporated in stabilization techniques (mainly arthrodesis) results in increased stress at the junction where the stabilized spine segment transitions to the nonfixed spine. Physiologic motion and/or gravitational force of the nonfixed portion will induce significant stress at this junction. The "stick-in-the-ground" provides a conceptual analogy. Hence, manual manipulation/bending of such a stick (fixed into the ground) will cause weakening and breakage at or near the junctional (ground) level. The precise level above ground of the induced stress is dependent on the flexibility of the stick, the extent of its fixation, and the site at which it is grasped.

Pathologically, postoperative junctional stress has two commonly recognized radiographic descriptions. (However, a spectrum of stress-related morphologic feature exists.)

- **Adjacent Segment Disease (ASD):** this refers to progressive and enhanced symptomatic degenerative change. Its special clinical relevance after *short-segment* stabilization constructs in PDLS surgery is to be determined, especially in regard to the interactive influences of underlying degenerative disease,[5] sagittal balance,[4] and obesity/paraspinous muscle morphology.[6] ASD affects the cephalad adjacent segment predominantly but not exclusively.[7] Symptomatically, it may present with primary axial

33

back pain and/or radicular pain from progressive stenosis at the next motion segment level above the fixed portion. Occasionally, it will be manifested at the second level above the stabilized spine. The potential for ASD is a function of the length of the stabilization construct.[8]

Kyphotic deformity and/or rotational instability can also be represented as junctional stress in the shorter stabilization constructs of PDLS surgery as a consequence of gravitational force (as per below).

- **Junctional Kyphosis:** this results most frequently after the longer deformity constructs employed in the treatment of adult degenerative scoliosis (ADS). It is a function of the motion of the unfixed spine and of gravitational force. The *sagittal rotational junctional stress* of gravitational force is a function of the mass on which it is exerted (i.e., essentially the body's weight above the junction) and of the horizontal distance of this mass from the junction (which is measured from the plumb-line through the gravitational center of the mass = its center of gravity). The term *kyphosis* refers to a sagittal rotation (one or more levels) which is essentially fixed. Thus, *junctional kyphosis* is a fixed segmental sagittal rotational deformity at the junctional level.

The concept of "balance" relates to the *potential* for creation of deformity rendered at the junctional region by the gravitational force (as described below); thus, the degree of imbalance is directly proportional to this potential.

4.4 Stabilization with Sagittal Imbalance

4.4.1 Relevance of SIB with Limited Stabilization of SFC Surgery

As noted earlier, SFC surgery is primarily concerned with radicular pain relief by decompressive surgical techniques. There is usually no attention to correction of deformity as a primary therapeutic directive. Some such correction often results from a needed stabilization procedure, but is limited segmentally. With an increasing knowledge of the role of an underlying *sagittal imbalance* (SIB) as etiological in the creation of pre- and postoperative symptomatic pathology, sagittal deformity evaluation has become more routine in the planning of SFC surgery on the PDLS.[9] This has particular relevance when stabilization instrumentation is otherwise indicated, as SIB can result in pathological stresses at the junctional regions of these constructs. In general, the longer the lumbar construct, the greater the potential pathologic stress rendered by SIB. Thus, sagittal balance evaluation may inform the surgeon as to the type and extent of any segmental stabilization planned. And, as such, it may be directive for a limited sagittal lordotic corrective maneuver at the index site or possibly at additional levels.

Although there is early outcome evidence of the need for addressing SIB, greater specificity of indications for lumbar lordotic enhancement in limited segmental stabilization remains to be established. Further clinical investigation will establish the determining interrelationship between balance evaluation technique, extent of SIB, length/type, and position of lumbar stabilization construct. Current recommendations are discussed in this chapter.

4.4.2 Relevance of SIB in Patients Not Requiring Stabilization

In patients not requiring stabilization, the specific imperatives for sagittal balance evaluation/correction have not yet been determined, although, in certain cases of multilevel decompression for lumbar stenosis, preoperative SIB evaluation may be important. There is evidence that laminectomy can, to a limited degree, improve sagittal parameters as a consequence of relieving the *compensatory* mechanism of a reduced lordosis, which provides claudication relief.[10,11,12] Those patients with a more significant SIB would not effectively be corrected by surgical decompression; with surgery, these patients may have claudication relief, but postoperatively they can develop persistent and progressive mechanical back pain (type unspecified). The potential for such postoperative pain may be relative to the extent of the surgical exposure, and may be minimized by microvascular decompressive techniques.[13]

However, in this subset of patients with lumbar stenosis, the specific indications for sagittal deformity correction need further clarification.

4.4.3 Relevance of SIB in Regard to the Potential Need for Osteotomy Techniques in SFC Surgery

The clinical/radiographic scenario(s) directing more aggressive SIB correction in SFC surgery for radicular pain of degenerative lumbar spine are currently not established. Further investigation is needed to determine if there are subgroups in the care of the PDLS that may require correction to the degree afforded by vertebral body osteotomy techniques. It is anticipated (by the author) that the complex multivariance in clinical presentation of the individual patient with the PDLS may prevent specific directives for complex sagittal correction. The advantage of any such sagittal balance gained must be weighed against the increased perioperative morbidity of these techniques within the framework of the individual patient with variant dysfunctional, comorbid, and psychosocial states.

4.4.4 Uncompensated SIB (Normal Pelvic Tilt [PT])[14]

Compensation for a measured abnormal sagittal alignment should be always be investigated. A normal PT, representing the absence of compensatory hip retroversion, should alert the physician to the possibility of hip flexion contracture, or of significant extensor muscle pathology. The latter can be either primary (degenerative flat back) or secondary (global decompensation). Also, patients with lumbar stenosis may initially lean forward in an attempt to reduce the lordotic root compression with an uncompensated global imbalance. However, they may eventually recruit compensatory mechanisms of balance compensation (pelvic retroversion, shift) as the desire of upright posture overrides that of neural compression.[12]

Therefore, when hip contracture and lumbar stenosis is ruled out in a patient with uncompensated SIB, then the risk for poststabilization failure is significant, usually accountable to extensor muscle functional deficiency.

Surgical planning in the correction of sagittal misalignment: In major scoliosis (deformity) surgery, the prediction of proper sagittal alignment correction (as measured by sagittal vertical axis [SVA]) has required mathematical formulation using LL, PI, and TK (thoracic kyphosis); and compensatory mechanisms which are age dependent. The most accurate of these is a complex equation that also uses PT and patient's age, thus factoring in retroversion compensation and the normal sagittal changes acquired in aging.[15]

Although major deformity correction is not within the realm of an SFC surgery on the PDLS, sagittal alignment may be pertinent in the situations when stabilization surgery is contemplated. Thus, in these situations (summarized at the end of this chapter), the surgeon must be able to evaluate the effect of limited sagittal alignment techniques with stabilization. There are several pertinent technical points in this regard.

- The lower (more caudal) any correction is made, the greater the effect on global balance. This is a function of triangle geometry: for any given angle formed by the equal sides of an isosceles triangle, the length of the third side is dependent on the length of the two equal sides. Any degree correction done at L5–S1 will geometrically yield the greatest change in the SVA or TPA (T1 pelvic angle), etc. However, other factors (e.g., thoracic reciprocal changes) can negate the geometric advantage of lower correction, to some degree.

- A relatively simple digital angular computation can give a rough assessment of the needed increase in segmental lordosis for global realignment (▶ Fig. 4.1).
- Stabilization techniques can reduce a compensated sagittal balance with negative consequences (e.g., the reduction at a low lumbar level of a "fish-mouthed" spondylolisthesis, with resulting normalization or parallelization of the end plate divergence, may have a significant negative effect on sagittal alignment).

4.5 Coronal Deformity Considerations

Midlumbar segmental deformity: Correction of coronal deformity in SFC surgery may be done secondarily as the consequence of stabilization for severe chronic axial lumbar and/or radicular pain. In cases of coronal collapse/tilt at an index (usually L3) level, a compensatory adult scoliosis may exist. Of significance is that correction of this segmental horizontal tilt may stop progression and induce correction of such compensatory scoliosis over time.[16] Hence, in cases of radicular pain from stenosis at the level of such midlumbar deformity with secondary adult *flexible* scoliosis (with or without significant axial pain), consideration must be given to segmental instrumented coronal correction. In all cases, flexibility and global coronal alignment must be determined. If the compensatory scoliosis is fixed, then segmental realignment may not be indicated.

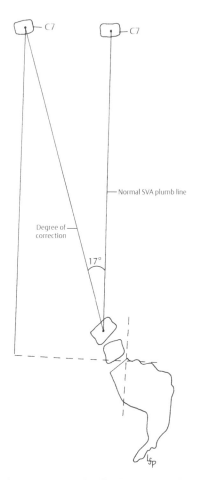

Fig. 4.1 Digital angular measurement for needed segmental sagittal correction.

Root compression at convexity of a coronal curve: If the coronal deformity is integral in symptomatic root compression, stabilization/limited correction may be indicated. Decompression of root(s) symptomatic by pedicle hooking at the concavity of a coronal curve would require limited corrective instrumentation/fusion to prevent worsening of the deformity and recurrence of radiculopathy.

Pelvic obliquity and leg-length discrepancy: A clinical and/or radiographic pelvic obliquity must be noted by the PDLS surgeon. This must be accounted for primarily: as secondary either to degenerative lumbar rotoscoliosis or to leg-length discrepancy.

The interrelationship between degenerative scoliosis, pelvic obliquity, and leg-length discrepancy may have relevance to the treatment of the presenting pain complaint. For instance, root decompression on the concavity of a scoliotic curve, with a shorter leg contralaterally, may provide pain relief only for limited time, and potentially worsen the scoliosis and/or lateral listhesis, if there is no attention to a primary leg-length discrepancy (shoe lift, hip arthroplasty).

These dynamics must be understood when there is indication for stabilization (see below). Currently, emphasis of sagittal balance correction in short-segment stabilization is focused on the occurrence of ASD.[4] However, there is frequently a pelvic obliquity and degenerative rotoscoliosis in the patient needing stabilization. The PDLS surgeon usually will consider addressing the coronal spinal deformity with targeted interbody placement or compression/contraction maneuvers. However, if this is done in ignorance of the primary driver of the pelvic obliquity (leg-length discrepancy), then the construct will undergo significant asymmetric stress, the overall coronal alignment may worsen,[14] and the effect on lumbar symptomatology may be limited or worsened.

4.6 SFC Surgery on the PDLS versus Adult Degenerative Scoliosis Surgery

With improved instrumentation for stabilization and deformity correction, there is a growing increase in the treatment of adults with significant degenerative deformity. Although many such techniques are common among SFC and ADS surgeries, the evaluative and operative differences are such that, presently, they should be considered as *separate clinical subspecialties* in the surgery on the degenerative spine. The obvious difference in these subspecialties is related to the anatomic extent of surgery required: SFC surgery on the PDLS is, by definition, essentially confined to the lumbar region (and upper sacrum); deformity correction in ADS surgery may require extension into the thoracic and cervical regions.

Another common technical point of division between SFC and ADS surgery relates to the capacity to provide extensive sagittal correction via three-column *osteotomy techniques.* However, if sagittal parameters assume greater relevance in surgery on the PDLS (as established by valid investigation), PDLS surgeons may adopt these aggressive osteotomy techniques with which more severe SIB patients can be corrected. Presently, posterior column osteotomies (PCOs) for more limited correction are in the PDLS surgeon's armamentarium.

Surgeons completing "Complex Spine" fellowships would address both PDLS and ADS entities. However, learning the nuances of proper PDLS surgery (as per this text) must begin in prefellowship training. Hence surgeons without a spine fellowship can effectively address limited stabilization in PDLS surgery.

4.7 Review of SFC for PDLS versus Deformity Surgery on the ADS

- Patient presentation:
  - PDLS surgery: radicular pain and/or severe axial segmental mechanical (antigravity) pain are the primary indications for surgery.
  - ADS surgery: radicular pain is often a key component; progressive deformity with functional and/or cosmetic sequelae; back pain symptomatology from deformity is usually more diffuse, not

truly axial (midline), and less segmental, representing muscular pain over scoliotic convexity; severe true axial segmental antigravity lumbar pain (CALPag) may be component of pain presentation

- Image evaluation
  - PDLS surgery: appropriate lumbar studies are done to assess suspected root compression or severe segmental degenerative pathology (i.e., in cases of severe chronic axial lumbar pain); secondary studies may be done to assess the need for a limited *adjunctive procedure with stabilization/sagittal correction* at the time of planned decompressive surgery; these include standing flexion-extension lateral plain films, scoliosis views for balance and pelvic parameter evaluation, and computed tomography (CT) scan to assess bony anatomy and/or degenerative stability. Coronal alignment and leg-length studies may be indicated with severe lumbar rotoscoliosis and/or evidence of pelvic obliquity.
  - ASD surgery: studies of the entire spine are usually required to plan appropriate deformity correction; these studies may be multiangular and/or digitally 3D reconstructed; *flexibility studies are an imperative*, including standing versus supine or prone comparisons, scoliosis films including the skull base and feet, global coronal plane analysis, Cobb's angle measurement of all curves, and measurement of sagittal cervical alignment
- Sagittal balance imperatives:
  - PDLS surgery: sagittal balance is evaluated in patients with *unstable* painful surgical pathology that requires fusion, in order to determine potential for postsurgical junctional stresses, thus dictating type and extent of corrective stabilization—or if in a patient having decompression for stenosis/claudication, it is to the extent that it may predispose the patient for postoperative

chronic back pain. In such situations, limited imbalance is addressed by positioning and/or expandable interbody cage and/or mechanical instrumentation manipulation. The PCO also is in the armamentarium of most PDLS surgeons. *It must be emphasized that the individual-specific clinical imperatives in these instances need further investigation.*

  - ASD surgery: major SIB correction is crucial for improved patient outcomes and may be addressed by three-column osteotomy techniques and extensive stabilization constructs. *The imperative for aggressive surgical correction of SIB with long instrumented constructs has been established in regard to the mechanical (junctional) and the clinical functional (e.g., ODI, HRQOL) advantage rendered.*[1,14,17]
- Coronal deformity imperatives:
  - PDLS surgery: some correction of coronal deformity may be done secondary to stabilization at a level of severe segmental axial mechanical (antigravity) pain. In unilateral root decompression surgery at a single level of midlumbar coronal collapse, instrumented segmental correction/stabilization may be indicated, as such tilt correction/fixation can reduce and/or reverse the compensatory curve on the unfused (flexible) main curve component in adult scoliosis.[16] A significant coronal curve may require consideration of limited stabilization if radicular pain is at the concavity of a scoliotic curve or if multilevel laminectomy for stenosis is anticipated at the center of the apex of such curve.[16] When stabilization is planned in cases of severe rotoscoliosis and/or pelvic obliquity, then coronal metrics need to be evaluated to determine need and extent of segmental deformity correction.
  - ASD surgery: correction of multiregional coronal deformity, as a result of lateral and rotatory instability, is primary and

is necessarily a major component in effectively addressing the patient symptoms and dysfunction resulting predominantly from the deformity and requiring extensive corrective instrumentation, the techniques and extent of which are dependent on flexibility studies.

4.8 Summary of Potential Indications for Limited Segmental Fusion/Stabilization in SFC Surgery on the PDLS

The potential for lumbar fusion techniques in SFC surgery are listed below. These will be discussed further in following chapters. It must be emphasized that these indications are relative to a thorough evaluation establishing any individual patient variables which would define risks precluding or limiting such surgery. Furthermore, as we increase our knowledge of fundamental and underlying mechanical factors, and their relevance to causation of symptomatic disease, these indications may be modified. *All general indications discussed may have patient-specific modifiers.*

1. When there is radiographic *instability* associated with the primary root compression symptomatology; or when there is a determined potential for progressive instability as rendered by the planned decompression procedure. This instability may or may not be associated with chronic antigravity axial lumbar pain (CALPag). The term "instability" does not have a uniform definition. It has most often been considered as a radiographic measurement of movement in standing flexion/extension lateral X-rays or standing versus supine images. The relevance of such motion is dependent on its degree and form within the clinical setting and operative needs of the individual patient.

2. When there is a severe and incapacitating *mechanical (antigravity) chronic axial lumbar pain (CALPag)* clearly associated with severe segmental-limited degenerative changes—either as the primary pain symptomatology or concomitant with significant root pain. (*Note: this indication for fusion remains controversial. See Chapter 9 for more extensive presentation.*)

3. When *sagittal alignment imbalance* (**SIB**) may result in anticipated abnormal junctional stresses for constructs in #1 and 2 above and thus requiring *additional* limited correction[4] or SIB may predispose a patient to chronic lumbar pain who is undergoing multilevel decompression for stenosis. (*Note: these indications are relative and patient specificity is not clearly established in the literature.*)

4. In adjacent segment disease (ASD), whether or not there is demonstrated macro-instability, thus requiring extension of instrumentation. (*Note: this indication is less controversial, although not absolute, and is individual-dependent.*)

5. In cases of **coronal scoliosis** when there is indication for root decompression at an index coronal tilt (L3 or L4) with secondary thoracic scoliotic compensation; or when root compression is a consequence of hooking deformity at the curve concavity.

4.9 Unknowns and Investigational Opportunities

- The relationship between the degree of SIB and construct length in determining potential for significant junctional stress after limited stabilization instrumentation in PDLS surgery.
- The relationship between SIB and the need for aggressive osteotomy techniques in PDLS surgery.
- The relationship between SIB and functional/pain results in patients having

5.1.1 Radicular Pain Evaluation

Historical Points

- **Discern as true radicular** symptomatology: note symptoms suggestive of nonradicular pain, or of the absence of dermatomal pattern or sensory symptoms, or of origination from lumbar region; if radiation only into buttocks, then establish para-axial lumbar origination.
- **Onset:** discogenic etiology most likely starting acutely.
- **Course**: length and severity—stable, worsening, improving.
- **Discogenic or stenotic** presentation: discogenic pain usually worse in sitting position; stenosis presenting with pain worse in upright position. If pain is worse in upright position, confirm *neurogenic claudication*: pain often severe in arising from chair; pain worse in walking up slight grades or stairs (occasionally worse walking down grades); pain relieved by sitting or bending forward. Mechanistically sitting stabilizes the pelvis, allowing the patient to reduce lumbar lordosis in a "slumping" posture. In the upright position, the patient can accomplish similar reduction in lumbar lordosis by anterior thrust of pelvis (hip extension/retroversion) and flexion of knees/ankles (▶ Fig. 5.1).
- **Motor symptoms** consistent with suspected root involvement: weakness of foot dorsiflexion or slap-foot ambulation (L5); or weakness in leg/knee going up stairs (L3/L4); weakness in hip flexion getting into car (L1, L2, L3).

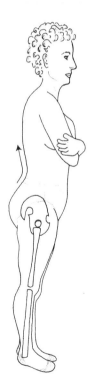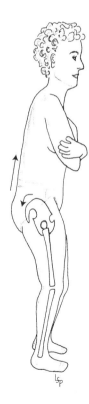

Fig. 5.1 Postural compensation for lumbar stenosis: pelvis retroversion and knee flexion to provide support and balance for forced reduction of lumbar lordosis.

Minimal Examination with Radicular Pain—Focused on Suspected Root(s) Involvement

- Lasègue (straight leg raise [SLR]): note degree bilaterally.
- Dorsiflexion weakness: extensor hallucis longus/foot.
- Deep tendon reflex (DTR) asymmetry in unilateral radicular pain syndrome: to confirm suspected root involvement (decreased patellar reflex [L4] and Achilles reflex [S1]).
- DTR in claudication syndrome: patellar–Achilles disparity supporting stenosis at L4–L5.
- **Important:** *active Achilles reflexes in symptomatic lumbar stenosis mandate focused myelopathic history/examination for symptoms and signs in upper extremities to rule out concurrent cervical stenosis.*
- Atrophy: calf (S1) and quadriceps (L3/L4).
- Ambulation: normal (for evidence of limp or hip waddle); toe-walking and heel-walking for evidence of nonphysiologic component, when suspected.
- Additional exam with suspected nonradicular or concurrent etiology: degenerative hip signs; sacroiliac joint (SIJ) or piriformis tenderness; pedal pulses (note: presence of one palpable pedal pulse does not exclude vascular pain).

Radiographic Studies

- Magnetic resonance imaging (MRI) is mainstay of radiographic confirmation of root compression—*consistent with root(s) involved as determined clinically.*
- Plain lumbar spine films:
  - Standard anteroposterior/lateral to assess for any unusual bony pathology or any anatomic variant.
  - Standing flexion/extension to assess for abnormal translational movement. Mandatory in patients with listhesis and/or stenosis.[1] And comparison of standing films with supine alignment (MRI or computed tomography [CT]).

5.2 Radicular Pain Presenting Predominantly in the Lower Back

Radicular pain can present with pain in para-axial lumbar region. This pain is not dermatomal but rather is dorsal rami pain via medial and intermediate branches (to facet and musculature). Thus, the common discogenic radicular pain from herniated nucleus within the spinal canal commonly radiates from this region. In contrast, spinal nerve pain from a lateral herniated nucleus pulposus will not present with para-axial lumbar pain.

Similarly, the radicular pain of lumbar stenosis often involves the para-axial lumbar spine and can be predominantly such. Hence, occasionally, patients with symptomatic lumbar stenosis will present with ambulatory/standing pain, unilateral or bilateral, in the para-axial lumbar area, sometimes radiating into the hips, but without overt leg pain (claudication).

5.3 Syndromes of Nonradicular Neurogenic Leg Pain

5.3.1 Piriformis Syndrome

Introduction

The piriformis syndrome remains a controversial diagnosis without consensus as to pathophysiology and diagnostic criteria. However, therapeutic results suggest that it is a bona fide clinical entity.[2] Injection therapy can result in a good response, sometimes with lasting benefit. And in refractory cases, surgical exploration/decompression also has been reported, in several studies, to have a success rate of about 80%.

History

- Pain emanating from buttocks *without* lumbosacral involvement.
- Pain worse with sitting.
- Possible dyspareunia in females.
- Possible history of trauma to buttocks—recent or remote.
- Pain predominantly of peroneal division of the sciatic nerve.

Examination

- Unequivocal tenderness at sciatic notch (most sensitive/specific).
- Straight leg raising—if positive, pain referred to buttocks (and not to lumbosacral spine).
- Provocative contraction of piriformis: resisted abduction of legs in seated position[3]; resisted abduction of flexed leg when in lateral decubitus position with asymptomatic side down.[4]
- Provocative stretching of piriformis: forceful internal rotation of extended leg[5]; forceful internal rotation with hip flexed and leg adducted.

Image Pathology

- Piriformis hypertrophy or abnormality (relative to asymptomatic side) on MRI or CT.
- Piriformis asymmetry/sciatic nerve hyperintensity on MR neurography.

Electrodiagnostic Pathology

- Delayed F waves and H reflex on nerve conduction studies (with external rotators tightened).
- Delayed somatosensory evoked potentials (at entry to buttocks) on nerve conduction studies.
- Electromyography (EMG) showing extrapelvic (nonradicular) compression.

Treatment

- Physical therapy: stretching, massage, and ultrasound, osteopathic manipulation.

- Guided injections: local anesthetic/steroids; botulinum type B.
- Surgical exploration.

5.3.2 Other Entrapment Neuropathies

Essentially, any peripheral nerve in the leg can be either entrapped or injured and thus become symptomatic. There are three relatively common symptomatic presentations which are referred to the PDLS surgeon, as they may resemble a sciatic symptomatic distribution. It is not difficult to differentiate these entities from more common radicular syndromes, but only when a dedicated symptom-focused evaluation is performed. A perfunctory history/exam in such a patient with an "abnormal" MRI will result in missed diagnosis and unnecessary and unsuccessful surgery.

Neuropathy of the Lateral Femoral Cutaneous Nerve[6]

Anatomy/pathophysiology: The lateral femoral cutaneous nerve is derived from posterior division of L2 and L3. Pathologic involvement occurs as it passes through the inguinal ligament just medial to the anterior superior iliac spine.

Symptomatology: Meralgia paresthetica is a common condition represented as hypesthesia/painful paresthesias of the cutaneous distribution of this afferent nerve. It does not have origin at the lumbar or buttocks region, and no symptoms should exist distal to the knee. In males, it is characteristically symptomatic by irritation from items in the over-lying trouser pocket and is often associated with a pendulous abdomen. In females, obesity also may precipitate it, or it may develop during pregnancy and persist after labor. Diabetes is the main comorbid factor as with any entrapment neuropathy.

Examination: Examination reveals hypesthesia in the characteristic distribution of the anterior/lateral thigh. There is usually asymmetric tenderness to deep pressure medial to the anterior superior iliac spine.

Therapy: Meralgia paresthetica is usually medically manageable (e.g., gabapentin) and is self-limiting. Rarely is surgery required. Its recognition by the PDLS surgeon will often save considerable diagnostic expense.

Neuropathy of the Common Peroneal Nerve[6]

Anatomy/pathophysiology: The common peroneal nerve (L4–S1) divides just distal to the fibular head into the deep and superficial branches. These, respectively, supply the dorsiflexors and evertors of the foot. Sensory distribution is to the dorsum of foot, usually sparing the fifth digit. The common pathologic compression at the fibular head usually spares the lateral cutaneous branch to the lateral calf.

Symptomatology: This neuropathy is usually associated with some history of compression: cast, legs crossed, occupational position, etc., and/or with some form of peripheral neuropathy. However, it rarely can occur de novo in an elderly patient. Here, it is usually more symptomatic with walking and can be misinterpreted as an L5 radicular claudication, especially with concomitant lumbar degenerative symptoms. However, the motor dysfunction (slap-foot, steppage gate) is out of proportion to pain symptomatology.

Examination: Dorsiflexion weakness may or may not be demonstrable, as symptoms often are intermittently related to walking or other activities. Asymmetric tenderness at the fibular neck is usually present. Palpation of popliteal fossa is important in presence of symptoms suggestive of involvement of lateral cutaneous branch at lateral calf.

Evaluation: Definitive diagnosis by electrophysiologic testing. With sensory symptoms representing lateral cutaneous branch, MRI evaluation of popliteal fossa

region indicated. Toxin screen (especially lead) may be indicated.

Therapy: Surgical exploration/decompression may be indicated when there is no acute compressive history and/or generalized peripheral neuropathy.

Neuropathy of Superior Cluneal Nerve[7,8,9]

Anatomy/pathophysiology: The superior cluneal nerve is a cutaneous afferent nerve deriving from the posterior rami of LI–L3. It perforates the thoracolumbar fascia just proximal to the ilium 7 to 8 cm from the midline supplying the skin of the lateral buttocks.

Symptomatology: Primary point of pain (PPP) described as radiating distinctly from ilium lateral to erector spinae at point of fascial perforation, radiating to lateral hip/thigh; without lumbar para-axial origin; usually worse with lumbar extension; often worse with walking and characteristically relieved by rest.

Examination: Tenderness at PPP with or without Tinel's sign.

Evaluation: Clinical diagnosis without specific diagnostics.

Therapy: Injection with local anesthetic/steroids reported to be successful.[10] Refractory cases may require surgical decompression.[11]

5.4 Nonneurogenic Leg Pain

5.4.1 Vascular Claudication

Introduction

Vascular leg pain/claudication is underdiagnosed by the spinal surgeon. It can present in a localized distribution suggestive of a dermatomal representation. It exists concomitantly in 25% of cases with neurogenic claudication. The surgeon should consider vascular evaluation in any patient with equivocal clinical–radiographic correlation for neurogenic claudication or with abnormal pedal pulse exam.

History (Suggestive of Vascular Etiology)

- Usually positive for other atherosclerotic arterial pathology and other risk factors (diabetes, hypertension, hyperlipidemia, smoking).
- Rarely involves lumbosacral or iliac areas.
- Claudication localized and nonradiating.
- Claudication usually distal to knee but can involve buttocks/thigh.
- No pain with standing or arising from chair.
- Without dermatomal sensory symptoms.
- Without subjective motor symptoms.

Examination

- Clinical evaluation has limited reliability in distinguishing vasculogenic claudication.[2,12,13]
- Attenuation or absence of pedal pulses (either dorsalis pedis or posterior tibialis) in only 60 to 70% of patients.
- Poor sensitivities of palpable attenuation of popliteal and femoral pulses preclude their value in examination.
- Noticeable palpable difference in temperature (cooler) of symptomatic side versus asymptomatic is significant.

Investigation

- Ankle-brachial index (ABI ≤ 0.9) sensitive screening test for presence of peripheral arterial disease (PAD).
- Exercise ABI for definitive diagnosis in patients with normal ABI.
- Toe-brachial index (TBI ≤ 0.6) has stronger association with severity of PAD symptoms than ABI.
- TBI recommended in patients with foot symptoms or severe diabetics, or as definitive study in elderly patients who cannot tolerate exercise ABI.

- Only about 50% of patients with abnormal ABI have vascular claudication; hence, abnormal ABI does not prove vascular etiology of claudication symptoms.
- However, a normal ABI essentially precludes vascular claudication (with symptoms above ankle).
- EMG protocol of paraspinous mapping may be definitive to establish neurogenic claudication in cases of questionable diagnosis.

Treatment

- All patients with abnormal ABI need vascular surgery referral (if ABI ≤ 0.5, then referral needs to be urgent) before lumbar surgery.
- In patients with lumbar stenosis with clinically consistent claudication, a normal ABI rules out concomitant vascular claudication.
- When neurogenic etiology for leg pain is not well defined in patients with normal ABI, more definitive studies for a vascular etiology (above) may be indicated.

5.4.2 Degenerative Hip Disease

Introduction

The pain of hip joint osteoarthritis may be difficult to distinguish from that from lumbar stenosis. And, not uncommonly, the two pathologic degenerative conditions coexist within the same patient, thus requiring prioritization of therapy.[14]

Anatomy

Innervation of the hip joint stems from L2 to S1 via ventral rami and their contributions to the femoral, obturator, sciatic, and superior gluteal nerves. This broad multilevel source of innervation would account for the manifold presentation of hip joint pain via pain-referral mechanism.

History

- Pain in the leg usually with hip pain in ambulating.
- Pain in groin and/or buttocks most prevalent but pain can exist in anterior and/or posterior thigh and anterior knee.
- Pain distribution is not restricted to above knee and may involve shin/calf.
- It can present with a lateral leg distribution, closely mimicking a stenotic L5 monoradicular claudication.
- Pain in bed with lateral recumbency and with the symptomatic side down is characteristic.
- Of note, there are rarely sensory symptoms reported (the existence of which would mitigate strongly in favor of a neurogenic etiology).

Examination

- Pain and restriction of motion with hip manipulation, especially with bent-knee thigh rotation (FABER test).
- Definite tenderness at posterior greater trochanter and/or groin.
- Observation of ambulation often reveals a distinctive waddle (when the patient elevates the diseased hip in order to rotate it forward).
- Testing for hip contracture: forced supine extension; the Thomas test.

Investigation

- Plain X-rays and CT scan will usually be appropriately positive.
- An MRI scan may be required when there is incongruency between the bony radiography and symptoms. (Note: avascular necrosis may be diagnosed only via MRI.)
- Diagnostic block of the hip joint is meaningful only if it yields an unequivocally positive response.
- A diagnostic block of L5 may resolve the hip pain (because of the dominant contribution of this nerve to joint innervation) and thus is not useful to distinguish hip joint pain from radicular claudication.

Treatment

- Referral to an orthopaedic surgeon.
- With evidence of concomitant symptomatic stenotic radiculopathy, initial root decompression will allow appropriate rehabilitation after hip surgery.

5.5 Chronic Pain Predominant in the Lower Back

5.5.1 Nonspecificity of the Term "Chronic Low Back Pain"

The **NIH Task Force** defined "chronic low back pain" (CLBP) as pain involving the area between the lower posterior margin of the rib cage and the horizontal gluteal fold (i.e., lumbar/sacral-coccyx/buttocks) which has been an ongoing problem for at least 3 months to the extent that it has been problematic for at least half the days over the past 6 months.[15] This definition has no anatomic specificity that is relevant to pathophysiologic processes. And yet hundreds of investigational articles have been published, and continue to be, concerning therapeutic intervention on this amorphous entity; all such publications are corrupted by the lack of clinical specificity.

Presently, the subclassification of CLBP is one the greatest imperatives in the science of spine care. There has been no substantial progress in this endeavor since the seminal paper of Bernard and Kirkaldy-Willis 30 years ago.[16]

The "problem" in chronic lower back pain classification has been well defined.[17] The legitimization of pain by diagnostic labeling has far-reaching ethical consequences. Such labels as "annular tear," "bulging disc," "facet pain," "discogenic," etc., are theories of pain etiology that are not subject to falsifiability testing and thus cannot be considered "scientific theory." In fact, diagnostic labels and etiologies are regularly falsified. Therapy (result) is not considered to have diagnostic value, and untestable hypotheses are used by practitioners to account for treatment failures: "poor technique," "poor patient selection," "psychosocial profile," etc. And, thus, the patient must bear this failure as a "difficult," "challenging," or "problem" patient. And, although the label has been falsified, the diagnosis is recirculated and used on the next willing and able patient.[17]

A recent study has subgrouped "nonspecific" lower back pain according to clinical course patterns (trajectories).[18] The documentation of such patterns would have more clinical relevance if they could be related to a greater specificity of symptom presentation. This could be provided by a subclassification system based on precise clinical description. *This is the fundamental step in eliminating the "nonspecificity" of lower back pain, and would establish a foundation for developing etiological and therapeutic investigation.*

5.5.2 Precise Clinical Description of Pain in the Lower Back

Precision of terms: the term "chronic low back pain" (and its acronym "CLBP") should be abandoned as it is not a clinical entity. It needs to be subclassified anatomically relevant to a specific area within the lower back. The acronymic "L" should refer to the "lumbar" area (and it will be done so in this book when used outside the use of the common non-specific term "CLBP").

Localization of the Primary Point of Pain (PPP) is defined as area of "worse pain" or where "pain starts" or "trigger point of pain" and localized by patient's hand and confirmed with the examiner's hand.
- *Area*: upper lumbar, midlumbar, lower lumbar; sacrum; coccyx; hip.
- *Laterality*: axial (midline); para-axial; flank (if lumbar area); medial hip (ilial);

central hip; lateral hip (femoral); inferior hip (gluteal fold).
- *Side/symmetry*: right; left; predominant side if bilateral.
- *Radiation* (precise description).

5.5.3 Specific Activity Causing Exacerbation of Pain

- *Lumbar flexion/compression*: sitting; bending forward (grossly or slightly as in standing at the sink).
- *Lumbar extension*: standing erect; walking, going up stairs; recumbency; reaching overhead.
- *Antigravity*: elevating from bent-over position; getting things off floor; getting out of chair.
- *Nocturnal recumbency* (note any specific position).
- *No specific exacerbating physical activity determined.*

5.5.4 Evaluation of Chronic Pain Predominant in the Lower Back

Historical Points

- Definition (see above).
- Precise localization of pain (see above).
- Mechanisms of exacerbation (see above).
- Onset and course (of progression or remittance).
- Secondary symptoms in hips/legs.

Examination

- Observe if patient has difficulty arising from chair to examining table.
- Extend/tilt patient to right/left to reproduce unilateral pain.
- **Grading scale for mechanical (antigravity) axial pain:** Flexion/re-erection: ask patient to touch toes with knees unflexed—note if any pain on flexion and grade antigravity pain (on re-erection):

- ○ Grade 0—patient re-erects without noticeable difficulty and denies any pain.
- ○ Grade 1—patient re-erects without noticeable difficulty but admits some pain (subjective pain).
- ○ Grade 2—patient re-erects with noticeable difficulty (slowly = objective pain).
- ○ Grade 3—patient re-erects with assistance (pushes on knees or furniture, etc.) (▶ Fig. 5.2).
- ○ Grade 4—patient has pain/muscle spasm in standing, will not attempt flexion, may have crutch or cane.
- Palpate PPP area (lumbar or buttocks) in prone position: in patients with anti-gravity pain, note any area/level of exquisite tenderness with fasciculations in midline to thumb pressure; in patients with focal unilateral pain, note focal area of tenderness to thumb pressure (vs contralateral asymptomatic side); in patients with primary buttocks pain, palpate primary pain site.

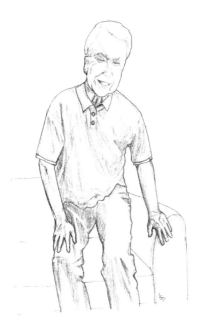

Fig. 5.2 Axial antigravity pain, grade 3: patient requiring assistance in elevating from seated or flexed position.

- Observation of normal ambulation.
- Provocative tests (hip, SIJ, piriformis) when pain not clearly from lumbar generator (see above for detail).
- Examination for leg-length discrepancy.

5.5.5 Chronic Axial Lumbar Pain (CALP)

There are two main forms of CALP. Clinically, either of these can be a primary complaint or may be associated with significant radicular symptoms.

Antigravity Chronic Axial Lumbar Pain (CALPag)

CALPag is the predominant presentation of "mechanical" pain. It is induced by activity of antigravity muscles, which are especially stressed in the attainment of a standing position from that of sitting, recumbency, or flexion. This form of CALP is prevalent and can be significantly incapacitating. Surgical evaluation/options are discussed in Chapter 8.

Compression-loading chronic axial lumbar pain (CALPcl)

Compression-loading pain is an uncommon indication for surgery in CALP. These patients represent a clinical/radiographic variation of the more common syndromes of symptomatic herniated discs. In distinction, however, the pain generator is primarily the posterior annular/posterior longitudinal ligament (PLL) complex, rather than the root. Mechanistically, this syndrome represents nociceptive stress transmitted through posterior nuclear displacement (case example in Blumenthal and Ohnmeiss[19]).

- History: Pain is described as primarily axial, but may have some radiation. It is characteristically worse with sitting or standing in slightly flexed position (as in washing dishes). It may have had distinct time and mechanism of onset, as with disc herniation. The pain often fluctuates in intensity.

- Exam: There are no objective findings other than possible paraspinous muscle spasm. SLR is equivocal or negative. On antigravity testing, the patient has greater pain in flexion (may be limited) than at re-erection not greater than grade 2.
- Radiographic/MRI: MRI reveals either general prolapse (soft) and/or subligamentous herniation(s). Disc height is normal or minimally diminished with T2 brightness.
- Surgical indication (after full course of "conservative" therapies): Distinct subligamentous extrusion/sequestration represents best indication as it allows for minimal surgical disc removal. In cases of general soft prolapse, nonopen techniques may provide a better option for limited excision of nucleus to reduce pressure on the posterior annulus/PLL, such as tubular microdiscectomy or intradiscal biaculoplasty.[20,21] (Note: the author has no experience with these techniques.)

5.6 Possible Infectious Etiology for Chronic Axial Pain of the Lumbar Spine

In the European literature, there has been emphasis on the concept of low-virulent anaerobic bacterial infection as the genesis for certain type of CLBP. The culture of herniated disc tissue has yielded positive results in as much as 70% of cases. *Propionibacterium acnes* appears to be the predominant organism in most studies,[22,23] though *Staphylococcus* has also been cultured.[24,25]

Modic type I change on MRI (bone edema) is postulated to represent a local inflammatory response to the adjacent disc infection. This is supported by a cohort study which establishes a relationship between the development of a postoperative Modic I appearance and positive disc cultures after herniated disc surgery.[26]

An elegant double-blinded randomized controlled trial[26] has studied the effect of long-term antibiotic treatment on patients with herniated lumbar disc and Modic I changes and CLBP of at least 6-month duration. These included both operated and nonoperated patients. In this study, 100 days of therapy with amoxicillin/clavulanate (500 mg/125 mg) yielded significant clinical improvement in all primary and secondary outcome measures, including sciatica. Of note is that many patients reported continued clinical improvement for a longer period. There was also a significant difference in the improvement in Modic I volume changes measured at 1-year follow-up.

This study appears (in some patients) to confirm an infectious etiology in CLBP associated with a specific Modic appearance (type I), and offers a potentially powerful conservative treatment option in this subgroup of patients. However, this relationship remains controversial. A recent Australian cohort study has emphasized the importance of contaminant controls needed to verify infection of disc material.[27] Patients with Modic type I changes and longstanding "CLBP" are also those which represent the best surgical candidates. Thus, further investigation is needed to identify subgroups relevant to potential response to either of these therapeutic measures. Furthermore, therapeutic consideration must allow for the frequent progression of Modic I changes to a more "stable" and less symptomatic Modic type II pattern.

In this study, "CLBP" is not subclassified in terms of location and activity of exacerbation (as per discussion above, it is assumed that this represents CALP). Such clinical specificity may help provide some predictive value in the identification of these subgroups: positive responders to antibiotics; negative responders requiring consideration of surgery; those that will progress in natural resolution to Modic type II changes.

The concept of low-virulent bacterial infection as etiologically significant in disc herniation and CLBP has other therapeutic implications. The role of intradiscal antibiotic therapy will necessarily be investigated. Similarly, there will be improvement in the techniques delineating the type and effects of varying offending infectious agents.

Inevitably, the conclusions of such investigations will affect the indications/techniques of surgical therapeutic intervention. For instance, the establishment of an infectious etiology (Modic type I) in a patient needing decompression for a herniated disc may influence the choice of microdiscectomy versus a more radical excision of the (infected) intervertebral disc. And if the patient has a significant component of axial mechanical pain (i.e., antigravity grade 3 or 4), then a concurrent stabilization procedure may be considered.

Finally, the investigations into the relationships between infection, chronic back pain, disc herniation, and radiographic images may lead to a greater understanding of the poorly understood mechanisms of lumbar pain generation and neural pain pathways.

5.7 Sacroiliac Joint Pain

In the recent several years, there has been a renewed increased interest in the SIJ as a cause of CLBP. A seminal paper by Schwarzer et al[28] established the existence of SIJ pain in an elegant study involving arthrography and double-injection blocks. This study was also placebo-controlled by the use of facet blocks.

This recent discussion has, in part, been engendered by the development of minimally invasive surgical (MIS) techniques for the fusion of the joint. Thus, industry-sponsored articles predominate in the literature currently. The value of these investigations/publications are recognized but must be tempered by the realization of their unavoidable bias.

Prevalence: The industry bias is clearly represented in their liberal publication of the prevalence of SIJ pain. One such industry-sponsored study[29] suggested the prevalence at 15 to 30% of "low back pain," and these numbers have been promulgated at an industry-sponsored course on MIS technique for SIJ fusion (author's experience). One of the references in support of this number was that of Schwarzer et al.[28] Yet, in this study, the group of 43 patients investigated had been preselected from a larger referral group of 100 patients, based on a pain presentation *below L5–S1*. In the larger overall group of 100, the prevalence of SIJ pain was 13%. Furthermore, these patients had been referred to the authors' radiology practice by outlying clinicians, and it can be assumed that these neurosurgeons, orthopaedists, and physiatrists had also added an initial selection process. Thus, based on this study, the prevalence of SIJ pain is likely less than 13% of patients with unselected low back pain presentation.

Thus, any prevalent statistic must clearly define the patient base investigated. Most diagnostic block studies have been done on selected patients with symptoms suggestive of pain caudal to the lumbar spine, and the prevalence rates of these studies vary. One study found an 18.8% rate in patients "… with a high likelihood of sacroiliac pain …."[30] Another study in a selected group of patients "… with suspected sacroiliac involvement …" found a rate of 10%. In the overall (unselected) group, the rate was only 2%.[31]

Thus, it may be concluded that, for those patients with primary symptomatology in the sacral/buttocks region and without other potential etiology, diagnostic SIJ block (s) would confirm the SIJ as the pain generator in 10 to 15% (at most). In all patients with "low back pain," however, this percentage would be considerably lower, likely less than 5%. There is considerable evidence that in the setting of previous lumbar fusion, especially of long constructs, the prevalence of SIJ pain is demonstrably higher.[32,33]

And it must be emphasized that the literature consistently shows a false-positive response of about 20% for diagnostic injections.[30,31]

(**Author's note:** These numbers of prevalence still seem extremely high. But I have no experience in surgical treatment of SIJ disease.)

5.7.1 Evaluation and Surgical Considerations

- Surgeons who take care of the PDLS occasionally see patients who have an incapacitating pain in the sacral/buttocks region and cannot attribute this pain to other pathology. Consideration of an SIJ etiology is warranted. The only surgical therapeutic option is SIJ fusion. With the development of MIS techniques, the impetus for SIJ fusion has increased, although risks may be higher than originally stated.[34]
- There are no features of historical, physical, or radiologic presentation, or their combination, that are absolute in establishing SIJ pain.
- The presence of groin pain in association with pain suggestive of SIJ etiology with sacral sulcus pain/tenderness may have diagnostic significance.[28]
- The absence of a characteristic pain when the joint is stressed in its natural function during ambulation is enigmatic.
- Provocative tests on examination may have discriminative power.[35] This consisted of a positive thigh-thrust and compression test along with one other positive maneuver: Gaenslen's test, Patrick's sign, and/or iliac distraction. When these tests are combined with the clinical reasoning process using the McKenzie evaluation, the diagnostic accuracy is enhanced.[36] Yet, the validity of these provocative tests has been established as "limited" in an extensive systematic review.[37]
- Radiographic evaluations are nondiagnostic. One study[38] subcategorized SIJ pain based on CT and/or X-ray. They designated "Sacroiliitis" when there was radiographic evidence of joint degeneration (and/or a history of prior fusion) and "SIJ Disruption" when there was asymmetric widening of the SIJs or contrast leakage during diagnostic block.
- The diagnostic joint block is considered the gold standard of diagnosis, but *it has no construct validity unless it is controlled.*[37] A positive response to block in most studies was established when there was at least a 70 to 80% pain reduction for a period of time, measured in hours.
- Injection therapy with anesthetic/steroids has been reported to have considerable long-term success in the SIJ pain of seronegative spondyloarthropathy.[39] Several studies have failed to duplicate this success in patients, although a more recent study[39] with the injection of triamcinolone acetonide has demonstrated a long-lasting efficacy in two-thirds of the patients with SIJ pain (without spondyloarthropathy) diagnostically confirmed with joint block. The mean of this duration was 36.8 ± 9.9 weeks. *Previous lumbar fusion was significantly associated with treatment failure, rendering only a 42% success rate.*
- Studies showing results of SIJ fusion (after SIJ block diagnosis) vary in reported success rate.[29] Only one of these was a controlled study.[26] The success rates were determined in varying ways, but the numbers suggest a 60 to 83% good/excellent response.
- Although MIS techniques have considerably reduced the complications of SIJ fusion, perioperative procedure–related events are significant (though eventually resolving) and were reported to be at 16.7%,[38] which included post-op medical problems.
- Postoperatively, patients are limited in weight-bearing (with walker or crutches) for minimum of 3 weeks.
- There are no long-term evaluative studies, and some long-term effects theoretically might be anticipated. The SIJ/ligaments is thought to dissipate stresses to the pelvic ring generated by the

mechanics of upright ambulation. Furthermore, there is ample evidence that these stresses are exaggerated in the presence of lumbar segmental fixation. With long fusion constructs extending to the sacrum, SIJ degeneration may be as high as 75%.[32] Thus, if fusion of the lumbar spine generates increased stress to the SIJ, then consideration must be given to reverse stresses to the lumbar spine generated by SIJ fusion. And as the SIJ rotates in ambulation (2%), the long-term effects to the contralateral hip joint must also be considered.

5.7.2 Conclusion

- Dysfunctional SIJ pain is a legitimate clinical entity presenting with sublumbar low back pain. It may be significantly prevalent in patients with long stabilization constructs ending in sacral fixation. Its de novo occurrence in patients without psychosocial distress or history of trauma is rare.
- A suspected clinical diagnosis should be corroborated by dedicated physical therapy evaluation (with expertise in provocative maneuvers and McKenzie's evaluative therapy).
- Long-acting anesthetic block (with 70–80% reduction response lasting hours) is the definitive diagnostic test. Only a series of anesthetic injections with placebo (saline) and/or controls (facet or hip injections) can be considered to have validity. Similarly, a series of therapeutic injections (anesthetic/steroids) with definite response (lasting weeks) should be considered as strongly diagnostic.
- A single diagnostic block has no validity.
- Surgery (fusion) should be considered the last-choice option in patients with refractory and dysfunctional SIJ pain as documented with vigorous controlled anesthetic block. A recent systemic review concluded that, although there is a subset of patients with SIJ pain for which surgery is beneficial, "…with the

difficulty in accurate diagnosis and evidence for the efficacy of SIJ fusion itself lacking, serious consideration of the cause of pain and alternative treatments should be given before performing the operation."[40]

5.8 Behavioral Assessment: Evaluation and Relevance of Psychosocial Factors

When you've suffered a great deal in life, each additional pain is both unbearable and trifling.

Yann Martel (Life of Pi)

As emphasized previously, surgery on the degenerative lumbar spine is done to relieve pain. The patient's experience of pain always encompasses both physiologic and psychological components in varying formulations of interrelationship. It is becoming well documented that preoperative measures of psychosocial distress is predictive, as an independent variable, of postoperative pain and functional outcome assessment.[41,42,43,44,45] Yet, there continues to be a lack of treatment in patients with psychiatric comorbidity.[46] In the general population, the lifetime prevalence of patients meeting criteria for a mood disorder is over 25%, and in those patients with chronic spinal pain, this percentage can be expected to be higher.[41]

Thus, for the surgeon who operates on the PDLS, the surgical decision-making process is often encumbered by psychosocial factors that have direct bearing on patient selection and/or on anticipated surgical results. Depression, especially, may be a negative prognostic factor.[47] In these instances, the surgeon must have the expertise and the appropriate evaluative data to define three broad groups of patients.
- Patients who have significant primary psychological suffering, without evidence

of definitive spinal pathology. The surgeon must avoid operation on these patients despite persistent pain complaints but insure that any suffering of these patients is otherwise optimally treated.

- Patients who have preoperative psychosocial distress, yet are clearly surgical candidates. These patients need to be provided with realistic postoperative goals and expectations and other strategies for improvement in lifestyle patterns. There is evidence that preoperative depression can be reduced by definitive surgical or effective nonoperative treatment.[48,49]
- Patients with evidence of psychosocial distress and questionable or equivocal indications for surgery. These patients often provide a difficult challenge to the surgeon who is trying to decide the probability of surgical success.

5.8.1 Three Categories of Psychosocial Factors (Often Interrelated):

- Mood and personality disorders: For the PDLS surgeon, depression and anxiety are frequently recognized as clinically relevant, especially in chronic pain syndromes.
- Cognitive/behavioral: This refers to the patient's perception of their condition and their pain. Patients who *catastrophize* magnify the effects of their condition to the point of helplessness. These feelings are carried over into the postoperative period with severe pain intensities and large analgesic requirements. "Kinesiophobia" may be associated with catastrophizing and refers to an extreme fear of movement or reinjury with avoidance of physical activity and other active coping strategies. These behavioral responses to pain also predispose to poorer surgical outcomes.
- Situational: These are factors well known to influence treatment outcomes especially when measured in terms of work

capability or timing to return to work. They include pending litigation, workman's compensation injuries, and job dissatisfaction. Lack of spousal/family support is another negative situational condition.

Clinical evaluative techniques: The surgeon should acquire available records of psychosocial factors and these should be noted. The current medication list, especially, will usually previse as to a significant mood/anxiety disorder.

In the examination room, the surgeon can further delineate the presence of these psychosocial issues in regard to the patient's current and specific pain complaint:

- *Affect*: The general demeanor of the patient is quite "depressed," without smiles and replete with negative responses.
- *Multisegmental and migrating complaints*: The patient presents with pain complaints not potentially attributable to a single etiology. Or, when the surgeon admits to diagnosis difficulty in one particular area, the patient will immediately engage the surgeon's attention to a separate pain complaint.
- *Insomnia*: The vast majority of these patients admit to a poor ability to sleep.
- *History of crying spells*: When asked, a positive response is always significant (albeit the patient will usually impute these episodes to "the pain").
- *Crying in the examination room*: When gently probed as to other "stresses," "worries," "personal losses," or "interpersonal issues," the patient may become tearful.
- *Direct questioning as to disability application*: If this is done as follow-up to question as to type of employment, the patient is usually unoffended and forthcoming.
- *Histrionics on examination*: It should be understood that a nonphysiologic examination commonly seen in situational psychosocial environment (above) can be nonvolitional, representing mood or cognitive/behavioral dysfunction.

- *Narcotic use*: depression and anxiety are associated with increased preoperative narcotic use.[50]

Formal assessment testing: provide qualitative and quantitative assessment of psychosocial distress:

- *Clinician-administered measurements* have limited usefulness as a routine screening technique in the spine surgeon's office.
  - The Structured Clinical Interview for the DSM-IV Axis 1 Disorders (SCID-1): this is administered by a behavioral professional specialist and is considered the "gold standard" for diagnosis of depression. However, its administration and scoring is lengthy.
  - Hamilton Rating Scale for Depression (HRSD).
  - Mental Health Component of Short Form Health Survey (SF-36), but it is proprietary.
- *Self-administered measurements* are easily administered and quickly graded and have significant evaluative utility for the spine surgeon.
  - Beck Depression Inventory (BDI).
  - Zung Depression Scale (ZDS).
  - Modified Zung Depression Index (mZDI).
  - Patient Health Questionnaire Depression Module (PHQ-9).
  - Modified Somatic Perception Questionnaire (MSPQ).
  - Distress and Risk Assessment Method (DRAM): components of MSPQ and the mZDI.[51]
  - Patient Reported Outcome Measurement Information System: PROMIS anxiety SF-4 and the depression SF-4.
  - SF-36 mental health scales: shown to be less accurate in determining depression than BDI and PHQ-6.[52]

5.8.2 Conclusion

- It is recommended that all patients fill out self-administered measurement

(note poor correlation between surgeon's clinical diagnosis of depression and actual measurement scores).

- Document that all patients with measurement of *major/severe* depression have (or have had) qualified psychological evaluation and regular follow-up.
- Group 3 patients (above) with *moderate* depression should see qualified health psychologist as part of surgical decision-making workup.

5.9 Unknowns and Investigational Opportunities

- Clinical trial of limited discectomy in cases of CALPcl.
- Investigation of pain generator and afferent pathways in CALPag.
- Extent/relationship of low-virulent disc infection in chronic axial lumbar pain.
- Role of paraspinal muscle insufficiency and/or mechanical disadvantage in the etiology of CALPag.
- Role of leg-length discrepancy in low back pain syndromes.
- Further development of simplified clinically administered screening psychometric evaluation in patients with low back pain syndromes.

References

[1] Segebarth B, Kurd MF, Haug PH, Davis R. Routine upright imaging for evaluating degenerative lumbar Stenosis. J Spinal Disord Tech. 2015; 28 (10):394–397

[2] Halpin RJ, Ganju A. Piriformis syndrome: a real pain in the buttock? Neurosurgery. 2009; 65(4) Suppl:A197–A202

[3] Pace JB, Nagle D. Piriform syndrome. West J Med. 1976; 124(6):435–439

[4] Beatty RA. The piriformis muscle syndrome: a simple diagnostic maneuver. Neurosurgery. 1994; 34(3):512–514, discussion 514

[5] Freiberg A, Vinke T. Sciatica and the sacroiliac joint. J Bone Joint Surg. 1934; 16:126–136

[6] DeJong R. The Neurologic Examination. 4th ed. Hagerstown, MD: Harper and Row; 1979

[7] Tubbs RS, Levin MR, Loukas M, Potts EA, Cohen-Gadol AA. Anatomy and landmarks for the superior and middle cluneal nerves: application to posterior iliac crest harvest and entrapment syndromes. J Neurosurg Spine. 2010; 13(3):356–359

[8] Strong EK, Davila JC. The cluneal nerve syndrome; a distinct type of low back pain. Ind Med Surg. 1957; 26(9):417–429

[9] Chiba Y, Isu T, Kim K, et al. Association between intermittent low-back pain and superior cluneal nerve entrapment neuropathy. J Neurosurg Spine. 2015; 24(2):1–5

[10] Talu GK, Ozyalçin S, Talu U. Superior cluneal nerve entrapment. Reg Anesth Pain Med. 2000; 25 (6):648–650

[11] Morimoto D, Isu T, Kim K, et al. Surgical treatment of superior cluneal nerve entrapment neuropathy. J Neurosurg Spine. 2013; 19(1):71–75

[12] Haig AJ, Park P, Henke PK, et al. Reliability of the clinical examination in the diagnosis of neurogenic versus vascular claudication. Spine J. 2013; 13(12):1826–1834

[13] Imagama S, Matsuyama Y, Sakai Y, et al. An arterial pulse examination is not sufficient for diagnosis of peripheral arterial disease in lumbar spinal canal stenosis: a prospective multicenter study. Spine. 2011; 36(15):1204–1210

[14] Saito J, Ohtori S, Kishida S, et al. Difficulty of diagnosing the origin of lower leg pain in patients with both lumbar spinal stenosis and hip joint osteoarthritis. Spine. 2012; 37(25):2089–2093

[15] Deyo RA, Dworkin SF, Amtmann D, et al. Report of the NIH task force on research standards for chronic low back pain. Spine. 2014; 39 (14):1128–1143

[16] Bernard TN, Jr, Kirkaldy-Willis WH. Recognizing specific characteristics of nonspecific low back pain. Clin Orthop Relat Res. 1987(217):266–280

[17] Shah RV. Spine pain classification: the problem. Spine. 2012; 37(22):1853–1855

[18] Kongsted A, Kent P, Hestbaek L, Vach W. Patients with low back pain had distinct clinical course patterns that were typically neither complete recovery nor constant pain. A latent class analysis of longitudinal data. Spine J. 2015; 15 (5):885–894

[19] Blumenthal S, Ohnmeiss D. Does surgery have a role in the treatment of patients with a Primary complaint of axial low back pain? The good, the bad, the ugly. SpineLine. 2016; XVII(3):24–28

[20] Freeman BJC. Efficacy of IDET and PIRFT for the treatment of discogenic low back pain. In: Szpalski M, Gunzburg R, Rydevik B, Le Huec JC, Mayer H, eds. Surgery for Low Back Pain. Berlin: Springer; 2010:95–100

[21] Desai MJ, Kapural L, Petersohn JD, et al. A prospective, randomized, multicenter, open-label trial comparing intradiscal biaculoplasty to conventional medical management for discogenic lumbar back pain. Spine. 2016; 41(13):1065–1074

[22] Stirling A, Worthington T, Rafiq M, Lambert PA, Elliott TS. Association between sciatica and Propionibacterium acnes. Lancet. 2001; 357 (9273):2024–2025

[23] Albert HB, Kjaer P, Jensen TS, Sorensen JS, Bendix T, Manniche C. Modic changes, possible causes and relation to low back pain. Med Hypotheses. 2008; 70(2):361–368

[24] Coscia MF, Denys GA, Wack MF. Propionibacterium acnes, coagulase-negative straphylococcus, and the "biofilm-like" intervertebral disc. Spine. 2016; 41(24):1860–1865

[25] Coscia M, Wack M, Denys G. Low virulence bacterial infections of intervertebral discs and the resultant spinal disease processes. Paper presented at: 38th Scoliosis Research Society Annual Conference; 2003; Quebec City, Canada

[26] Albert HB, Sorensen JS, Christensen BS, Manniche C. Antibiotic treatment in patients with chronic low back pain and vertebral bone edema (Modic type 1 changes): a double-blind randomized clinical controlled trial of efficacy. Eur Spine J. 2013; 22(4):697–707

[27] Rao PJ, Phan K, Reddy R, Scherman DB, Taylor P, Mobbs RJ. DISC (degenerate-disc infection study with Contaminant control). Spine. 2016; 41 (11):935–939

[28] Schwarzer AC, Aprill CN, Bogduk N. The sacroiliac joint in chronic low back pain. Spine. 1995; 20 (1):31–37

[29] Rudolf L. Sacroiliac joint arthrodesis-MIS technique with titanium implants: report of the first 50 patients and outcomes. Open Orthop J. 2012; 6:495–502

[30] Maigne J-Y, Aivaliklis A, Pfefer F. Results of sacroiliac joint double block and value of sacroiliac pain provocation tests in 54 patients with low back pain. Spine. 1996; 21(16):1889–1892

[31] Manchikanti L, Singh V, Pampati V, et al. Evaluation of the relative contributions of various structures in chronic low back pain. Pain Physician. 2001; 4(4):308–316

[32] Schroeder JE, Cunningham ME, Ross T, et al. Early results of sacro-iliac joint fixation following long fusion to the sacrum in adult spine deformity. Available at: http://dx.doi.org/doi:10.1007/s11420-013–9374–4. Accessed May 5, 2015

[33] Unoki E, Abe E, Murai H, Kobayashi T, Abe T. Fusion of multiple segments can increase the incidence of nsacroiliac joint pain after lumbar or lumbosacral fusion. Spine. 2016; 41 (12):999–1005

[34] Schoell K, Buser Z, Jakoi A, et al. Postoperative complications in patients undergoing minimally invasive sacroiliac fusion. Spine J. 2016; 16 (11):1324–1332

[35] Szadek KM, van der Wurff P, van Tulder MW, Zuurmond WW, Perez RSGM. Diagnostic validity of criteria for sacroiliac joint pain: a systematic review. J Pain. 2009; 10(4):354–368

[36] Laslett M, Young SB, Aprill CN, McDonald B. Diagnosing painful sacroiliac joints: A validity study of a McKenzie evaluation and sacroiliac provocation tests. Aust J Physiother. 2003; 49(2):89–97

[37] Hansen HC, McKenzie-Brown AM, Cohen SP, Swicegood JR, Colson JD, Manchikanti L. Sacroiliac joint interventions: a systematic review. Pain Physician. 2007; 10(1):165–184

[38] Whang P, Cher D, Polly D, et al. Sacroiliac joint fusion using triangular titanium implants vs. nonsurgical management: six-month outcomes from a prospective randomized controlled trial. Int J Spine Surg. 2015; 9:6

[39] Liliang P-C, Lu K, Weng H-C, Liang C-L, Tsai Y-D, Chen H-J. The therapeutic efficacy of sacroiliac joint blocks with triamcinolone acetonide in the treatment of sacroiliac joint dysfunction without spondyloarthropathy. Spine. 2009; 34(9):896–900

[40] Zaidi HA, Montoure AJ, Dickman CA. Surgical and clinical efficacy of sacroiliac joint fusion: a systematic review of the literature. J Neurosurg Spine. 2015; 23(1):59–66

[41] Van Dorsten B, Lindley E. Improving outcomes via behavioral assessment of spine surgery candidates. SpineLine. 2010; XI(1):15–20

[42] Miller JA, Derakhshan A, Lubelski D, et al. The impact of preoperative depression on quality of life outcomes after lumbar surgery. Spine J. 2015; 15(1):58–64

[43] Chaichana KL, Mukherjee D, Adogwa O, Cheng JS, McGirt MJ. Correlation of preoperative depression and somatic perception scales with postoperative disability and quality of life after lumbar discectomy. Available at: http://dx.doi.org/DOI:10.3171/2010.10.SPINE10190. Accessed May 5, 2015

[44] Adogwa O, Parker SL, Shau DN, et al. Preoperative Zung Depression Scale predicts outcome after revision lumbar surgery for adjacent segment disease, recurrent stenosis, and pseudarthrosis. Spine J. 201 2; 1; 2(3):175–185

[45] Anderson JT, Haas AR, Percy R, Woods ST, Ahn UM, Ahn NU. Clinical depression is a strong predictor of poor lumbar fusion outcomes among workers' compensation subjects. Spine. 2015; 40 (10):748–756

[46] Konnopka A, Heinrich S, Zieger M, et al. Effects of psychiatric comorbidity on costs in patients undergoing disc surgery: a cross-sectional study. Spine J. 2011; 11(7):601–609

[47] Pinheiro MB, Ferreira ML, Refshauge K, et al. Symptoms of depression as a prognostic factor for low back pain: a systematic review. Spine J. 2016; 16(1):105–116

[48] Urban-Baeza A, Zárate-Kalfópulos B, Romero-Vargas S, Obil-Chavarría C, Brenes-Rojas L, Reyes-Sánchez A. Influence of depression symptoms on patient expectations and clinical outcomes in the surgical management of spinal stenosis. J Neurosurg Spine. 2015; 22(1):75–79

[49] Lubelski D, Thompson N, Bansal SK, et al. Depression predicts worse quality of life outcomes following nonoperative treatment for lumbar stenosis. Spine J. 2014; 14(11):48–49

[50] Armaghani SJ, Lee DS, Bible JE, et al. Preoperative narcotic use and its relation to depression and anxiety in patients undergoing spine surgery. Spine. 2013; 38(25):2196–2200

[51] Hung M, Stuart A, Cheng C, et al. Predicting the DRAM mZDI using the PROMIS anxiety and depression. Spine. 2015; 40(3):179–183

[52] Choi Y, Mayer TG, Williams MJ, Gatchel RJ. What is the best screening test for depression in chronic spinal pain patients? Spine J. 2014; 14(7):1175–1182

6 The Fundamental Open Surgical Method

Abstract

Considerable experience in open techniques is necessary before the PDLS surgeon can learn the nuances of pathological anatomy and its appropriate operative therapy. However, if certain technical fundamentals are appreciated, this experience will be rendered efficiently and safely.

The most common procedure for the PDLS surgeon is unilateral root decompression. A step-by-step routine for this exposure (as described) is important, though an uncompromising allegiance to it is not recommended. This technique can be expanded to gain visual and manual access for decompression of the contralateral side, with preservation of the laminae. When foraminal or extra-foraminal root decompression is needed, this can be done with or without preservation of the pars.

The (total) hemilaminectomy from caudal to cephalad is a safe and versatile technique when unilateral root compression pathology is complex. It also can be expanded medially to allow contralateral decompression in selected patients.

In severe cases of severe and multilevel stenosis, complete laminectomy is usually the safest and most effective technique. The "en bloc" laminectomy technique has been developed and allows the surgeon a margin of safety from dural disruption beyond that of the common piecemeal laminectomy.

Root decompression in operated anatomy can present a challenge. With cicatrix present, the surgeon must always effect the necessary exposure at the lateral margin of the spinal canal (medial to the facets). Decompression of any residual compression must proceed lateral to medial.

Placement of pedicle screws for arthrodesis requires precise fluoroscopic guidance as there is individual variance of pedicle entry vis-a-vis landmarks. Iliac fixation is rarely necessary in PDLS surgery; the S2 alar technique has some advantages over that of the more common iliac screws fixation.

Keywords: en bloc laminectomy, U-turn technique, parsectomy, extra-foraminal, lateral corridor, S2 alar iliac screw, shoe-string dural closure

One thing alone not even God can do, to make undone whatever hath been done.

Aristotle

We are what we repeatedly do. Excellence, then, is not an act, but a habit.

Aristotle

6.1 Introduction

Although the pathophysiologic processes in surgical PDLS are few, the individual pathological anatomy is multiplex. For instance, magnetic resonance imaging (MRI) depiction of a herniated lumbar disc may be unequivocal, and yet the surgeon will not gain from its review other important specifics to be determined only by direct operative visualization. Is the herniation contained, or partially or completely extruded? Is the posterior longitudinal ligament attenuated or is it essentially intact with a small defect? Has there been significant annular disruption? Is there herniated disc in the root axilla? Is there potential for residual interspace disc to extrude? And if pathology is recurrent with previous surgery, the surgeon cannot anticipate from the MRI the precise extent of the cicatrix, adhesions, and dural thinning. Furthermore, anomalous root pathology is not infrequent and usually is unappreciated on the MRI.

Such information can be crucial to the success of the surgery on a short- and long-term basis. Open operative techniques allow for maximal intraoperative assessment and instrument manipulation. Minimally invasive surgery on the PDLS has wide acceptance. However, its application requires a surgeon who is experienced in open techniques. *Without such experience, the nuances of anatomy and pathology cannot be learned effectively.*

Thus, the open methods described in this chapter will give the young surgeon the safest and most educational experience in the operating room. They are applicable to the full gamut of PDLS pathology.

6.2 Surgical Decision-Making Processes

6.2.1 Patient–Surgeon Interaction in Surgical Decision-Making

- Degenerative lumbar spine surgery (99%) is for subjective symptom (pain) relief and thus the patient must have significant input into surgical decision-making.
- With rare exception, no patient "needs" surgery to prevent significant neurological compromise (exceptions are patients with: a cauda equina syndrome; painful progressive foot-drop; painful progressive quadriceps weakness).
- If pain symptomatology is improving, then surgical decision should be deferred.
- If the patient decides he/she "can live with the pain," this is not to be discouraged.
- Risks of surgery, including those from comorbidities, should be clearly explained and documented.
- Follow-up evaluation may be necessary before the surgeon (and the patient) can make the appropriate decision.

6.2.2 Operative Plan with Radicular Pain Presentation

- Surgeon's mission: as limited decompression as possible.
- Identification of image pathology consistent with radicular pain syndrome.
- Indistinct correlation between clinically symptomatic root(s) and image may require extension of decompression.
- Prophylactic decompression for asymptomatic image pathology, while addressing the symptomatic level, is decided on an individual basis.
- No attention to correction of deformity unless relevant to root decompression— actually or potentially.
- Instrumentation avoided without clear indication.

6.2.3 Operative Plan with Primary Axial Lumbar Pain

- Operative treatment remains controversial.
- Compression-loading chronic axial lumbar pain (CALPcl) from disc prolapse or posterior subligamentous herniation) may rarely require limited discectomy.
- In the setting of high-grade anti-gravity chronic axial lumbar pain (CALPag), best surgical candidate is with severe degenerative discogenic/interspace changes (with bone edema) on MRI (with/without listhesis) at a single level.
- Positive disc-block response would provide further weight to selective process. If a repeat of a negative disc-block remains unchanged, then surgery is not indicated.
- Dynamic standing flexion-extension X-rays should be evaluated for abnormal motion (especially hyperrotation) at levels that appear normal on MRI.

- Therapeutic arthrodesis at painful level at discretion of surgeon (bony arthrodesis with/without various instrumentation options is most common); nonbony "dynamic" arthrodesis can provide a clinically effective stability.
- Reduction of listhesis at painful level may be detrimental in terms of hardware stress and effect on sagittal alignment.
- Multilevel degenerative changes on MRI are problematic for determining painful level and/or for increased potential of developing symptomatic adjacent segment disease; the resulting long-term risk–return ratio is thus negatively affected.

6.3 Fundamentals

6.3.1 Opening and Closure of Surgical Incision

- The length of the skin incision is only relevant if it is too small and thus hindering visualization and/or manipulation of instruments.
- The deep fascia is cleared bilaterally to allow for layered anatomic closure.
- At closure, meticulous attention to epidural and muscular wall hemostasis will obviate the need for a drain in most cases.
- Closure of the fascia is done with interrupted sutures. For easier anatomic closure, it is recommended that all fascial sutures be placed before tying them down.
- Optional attachment of fascia to spinous process (SP; ▶ Fig. 6.1).
- Closure of subcutaneous adipose tissue adds some element of strength resisting wound dehiscence, especially in obese patients.
- Superficial subcutaneous closure (inverted absorbable suture) of the

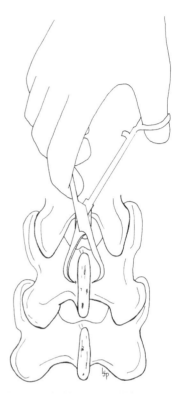

Fig. 6.1 Augering spinous process with towel clip for anatomic closure of deep fascia.

dermis is imperative in establishing an adequate well-apposed skin closure.
- Any drainage catheter should exit cephalad to incision, away from fecal contamination.

6.3.2 Decompression with Nonoperated Anatomy

- The ligamentum flavum is preserved as much as possible during primary bone removal, thus serving as a barrier of safety preventing durotomy.

- The ligamentum flavum is always removed by detaching it laterally (with Kerrison rongeurs) beginning at either its upper (cephalad) or lower (caudal) edge. It will thus be separated from underlying dura in a lateral-to-medial fashion. Complete removal requires its medial incision (near midline) before or after lateral detachment.
- Early nerve root visualization is done, whenever possible, before attention to its compressive pathology. With intracanalicular pathology, this visualization is almost always distal to the pathology (i.e., foraminal entrance).

6.4 Unilateral Decompression of Nerve Root with Nonoperated Anatomy: The "U-Turn" Technique

This is the fundamental root decompression technique for common pathologies with normal (nonoperated) anatomy.

6.4.1 Clinical Presentation

- Unilateral congruent monoradiculopathy (discogenic or stenotic).

6.4.2 Image Pathology

- Herniated lumbar disc.
- Subarticular (lateral recess) stenosis on symptomatic side.
- Small/moderate synovial cyst.

6.4.3 Contraindication

- Moderate/severe central stenosis (with thick hypertrophic ligamentum flavum).
- Large synovial cyst extending to midline.

6.4.4 Operative Procedure

(After surgeon's preference for positioning, skin prep, localization.)

1. Incision through deep fascia with cautery to expose SP and lamina of cephalad (superior) and caudal (inferior) vertebrae.
2. Subperiosteal dissection with cautery laterally from lamina along medial inferior articular process (IAP) of superior vertebra to drop-off into medial facet space.
3. Clearance of lamina and medial pars of inferior vertebra.
4. Begin partial hemilaminectomy of superior lamina by rongeuring (Leksell) its lower edge.
5. Drilling to expand partial hemilaminectomy and extending laterally along medial aspect of IAP (approximately 3 mm).
6. Completion of partial hemilaminectomy to upper edge of ligamentum flavum with Kerrison rongeurs confirmed by visualization of dura and/or epidural adipose tissue (▶ Fig. 6.2).
7. Extension of bone removal with Kerrison rongeurs laterally along medial aspect of IAP *external to* ligamentum flavum and extending to facet.
8. Grasping superficial leaf of ligamentum flavum and its removal from medial facet and inferior laminal attachment, with visualization of deep leaf attachment under cephalad edge of inferior lamina.
9. Beginning U-turn epidural decompression by lifting medial/superior edge of ligamentum flavum (under superior lamina) with nerve hook and inserting underneath a 1- or 2-mm Kerrison for its incision medially/caudally to inferior lamina (▶ Fig. 6.3).
10. With 2- or 3-mm Kerrison, advancing laterally (footplate heel medial) removing

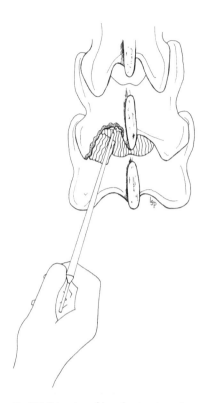

Fig. 6.2 Extension of hemilaminectomy to above attachment of ligamentum flavum.

upper edge of inferior lamina to pars, and visualization of root at entrance to foramen (distal to pathology) (▶ Fig. 6.4).

11. Continuing cephalad grasping ligamentum flavum laterally until complete removal. (Important: if root has not been visualized, then the surgeon may be distal to foraminal exit of root and thus must be careful advancing cephalad until root anatomy established.) (▶ Fig. 6.5).

(Note: The surgeon may elect to remove ligament from cephalad lateral edge caudally, when pathology is nonadherent to dorsal aspect of root: cicatrix, synovial cyst.)

12. Follow-up extension of foraminotomy and further lateral decompression as necessary using drill/Kerrison.

6.4.5 Alternative Process of Gaining Epidural Access (Best at L5–S1)

Steps 1 to 8 above, followed by:

- Using Kerrison to remove upper edge of inferior lamina by pressing ligamentum flavum down away from its attachment and visualizing epidural space (▶ Fig. 6.6).
- Incision of ligamentum flavum medially with 1-mm Kerrison working cephalad, and then continuing with larger Kerrisons laterally with detachment/incision of ligament from superior lamina and pedicle (▶ Fig. 6.7).
- May then continue removing ligament cephalad-to-caudal along axis of root or revert back to steps 10 to 12 above (see ▶ Fig. 6.4).

6.5 Bilateral Decompression by Direct Approach on One Side (U-Turn) and Then Contralateral Decompression under Interspinous/ Supraspinous Ligaments (Surgeon Working from One Side)

6.5.1 Clinical Presentation

- Unilateral or bilateral congruent stenotic monoradiculopathy(s).

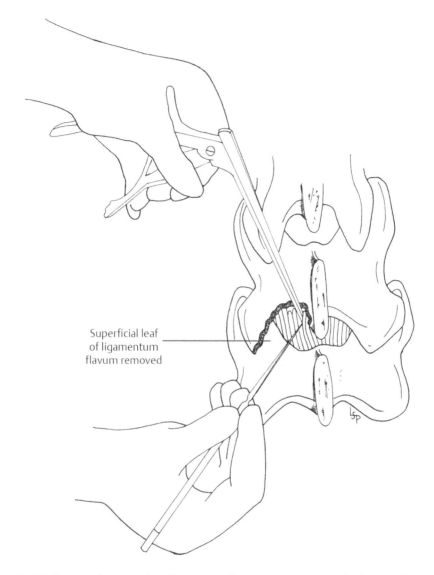

Superficial leaf
of ligamentum
flavum removed

Fig. 6.3 Elevation of superior edge of ligamentum flavum to gain access to epidural space to begin medial arm of U-turn, with extension of ligamentum incision caudally to under lamina edge.

6.5.2 Image Pathology

- Bilateral nonlisthetic subarticular (lateral recess) stenosis (one or multiple levels).
- Spondylolisthesis.[1]

6.5.3 Contraindications

- Severe/moderate central stenosis with hypertrophic ligamentum flavum.

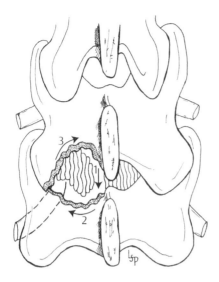

Fig. 6.4 Visualization of root at foramen at bottom of U-turn.

6.5.4 Operative Technique

1. Unilateral root decompression as above with modification:
   - Extension of step #1 above to gain visual access across midline by either of the following:
     a) Using cautery to expose midline edges of opposing SPs and thus cauterizing back interspinous ligament. May extend to expose medial edges of contralateral laminae.
     b) More aggressively by taking down muscle attachment from contralateral SPs and medial laminae and rongeuring away interspinous ligament and adjacent parts of SPs.
   - Extension of step #4/5 by drilling back (or rongeuring/drilling) both of these contralateral laminar edges and area of their junction with laminae.
2. Angling Kerrisons across midline to remove ligamentum flavum and facet edges for decompression. A small #7 suction (multi-perforated) is used for

visualization by downward compression of dura (▶ Fig. 6.8).

6.6 Bilateral Cross-Decompression with Removal of Interspinous/ Supraspinous Ligaments (Surgeon Working from Both Sides)

6.6.1 Clinical Presentation, Image Pathology, and Contraindications

As per previous section.

6.6.2 Operative Technique

1. Bilateral exposure of SPs and laminae.
2. Removal of interspinous ligament with cautery (or Leksell rongeur) (▶ Fig. 6.9).

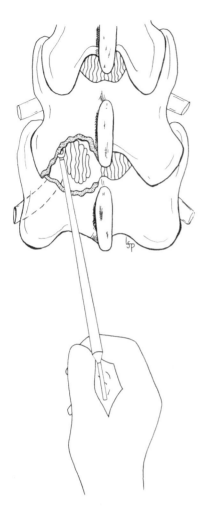

Fig. 6.5 Advancing cephalad with removal of ligament/medial facet in lateral arm of U-turn.

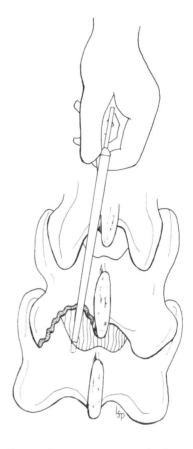

Fig. 6.6 Alternative access to epidural space under inferior lamina—most effectively used at L5–S1 and in reoperations.

3. Rongeuring or drilling of apposed SP edges as necessary.
4. Removal of bone (drilling/rongeur) bilaterally off laminar edges and IAPs *external to ligament*.
5. By cross-cutting, removal of cephalad edge of lower lamina, working laterally, and identifying caudal edge of ligament (▶ Fig. 6.10).

6. Continuing cephalad with lateral under-cutting decompression.
7. From opposite side of table, repeat process.

6.7 Laminectomy(s) by Piecemeal Rongeuring

6.7.1 Clinical Presentation

- Neurogenic claudication (unilateral or bilateral).

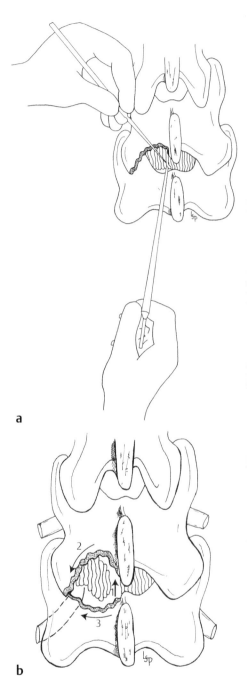

Fig. 6.7 (a) Medial incision of ligament advancing cephalad. **(b)** Advancing superolaterally for detachment of ligamentum flavum at pedicle.

a

b

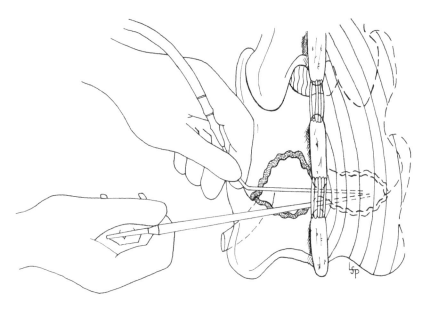

Fig. 6.8 Interspinous cross-cutting decompression after direct ipsilateral decompression.

6.7.2 Image Pathology

- Single or multilevel severe/moderate central stenosis with significant ligamentum flavum hypertrophy.

6.7.3 Contraindications

- None.

6.7.4 Operative Technique

1. Bilateral exposure to include medial facet space at each level with removal of superficial leaf of ligamentum flavum's facet attachment.

2. Optional drilling/rongeuring along medial IAP at each level.
3. Removal of SPs with rongeur (all levels or sequentially).
4. Creating 3- to 4-mm medial laminectomy at each level—advancing cephalad and remaining *external to ligamentum flavum* (to upper edge) at each level (▶ Fig. 6.11).
5. Further bone removal as necessary by drilling/rongeuring external to ligamentum flavum.
6. Final bilateral removal of ligamentum flavum (ipsilaterally and/or contralaterally via cross-cutting) for root visualization and decompression: identifying

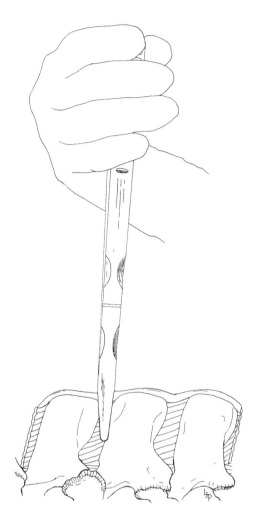

Fig. 6.9 Surgical site preparation for bilateral cross-cutting decompression.

caudal and cephalad edge at each level and stripping it from its lateral attachment by advancing with Kerrisons (angled 45 degrees inward) along lateral wall and thus peeling ligamentum flavum from dura in *lateral-to-medial* fashion (▶ Fig. 6.12).

6.8 Laminectomy(s) by En Bloc Technique

6.8.1 Introduction

This technique is now used exclusively by the author for total laminectomy(s). It is

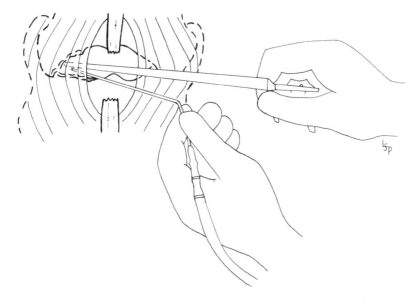

Fig. 6.10 Visualization across midline and access to inferior edge of ligamentum overlying root.

the safest technique in that it provides a one-step bony removal process, leaving the ligamentum flavum intact; thus, dural decompression from ligament/adhesions is clearly visualized and manipulated.

6.8.2 Clinical Presentation

• Neurogenic claudication (unilateral or bilateral).

6.8.3 Image Pathology

• Single or multilevel moderate or severe central stenosis with significant ligamentum flavum hypertrophy.

6.8.4 Contraindications

• None.

6.8.5 Operative Technique

1. Bilateral exposure to include medial facet space at each level with removal (by cauterizing back) of superficial leaf of ligamentum flavum and *to include visualization of upper edge of laminae* (note: preparation for en bloc removal can be done one side at a time).
2. Optional drilling along medial IAP at each level.
3. Development of plane between posterior lamina and ligamentum flavum.
4. Using drill (matchstick burr) to score/thin-out lamina, making thin trough from upper/medial to lower edge (▸ Fig. 6.13a).
5. Incise lamina along resulting trough with 2-mm Kerrison, remaining external to ligamentum flavum throughout

69

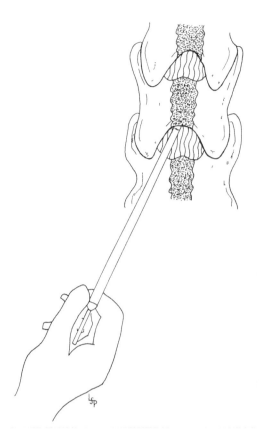

Fig. 6.11 Beginning piecemeal laminectomy after removal of spinous processes.

its laminal attachment, and then continue cephalad by widening trough above facet (secondary drilling as necessary); continue until Kerrison is completely through lamina (grabbing only ligament) (▶ Fig. 6.13b).

6. Incision of interspinous ligament at each end of decompression.

7. En bloc removal of SPs/medial laminae by lifting (Leksell rongeur) most caudal level and peeling it in cephalad direction. If intervening interspinous ligaments are intact, entire medial decompression is removed in one piece (▶ Fig. 6.14).

8. Cross-cutting lateral decompression with removal of additional bone (as needed) and ligamentum flavum by undercutting, advancing longitudinally with Kerrisons starting at upper and/or lower edge at its lateral attachment and stripping ligamentum flavum lateral to medial; visualization of each exiting root or its surrounding adipose tissue (▶ Fig. 6.15).

6.9 Hemilaminectomy (s): Versatility and Safety

6.9.1 Introduction

Hemilaminectomy has universal application for neural decompression. It provides

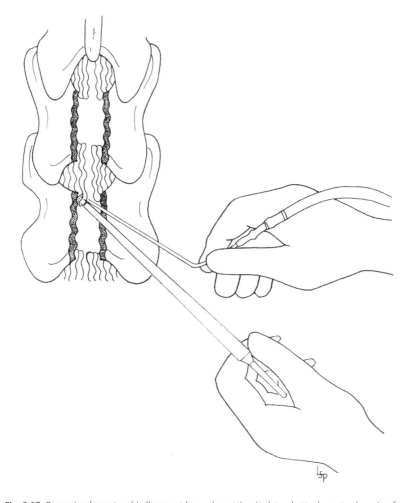

Fig. 6.12 Removing hypertrophic ligament by undercutting its lateral attachment advancing from cephalad and/or caudal edge.

optimal safety in entering the spinal canal and thus has special application in delicate surgical situations and those with unusual and/or difficult pathologies.

6.9.2 Clinical Presentation

• Painful radiculopathy—unilateral or bilateral, discogenic and/or stenotic.

71

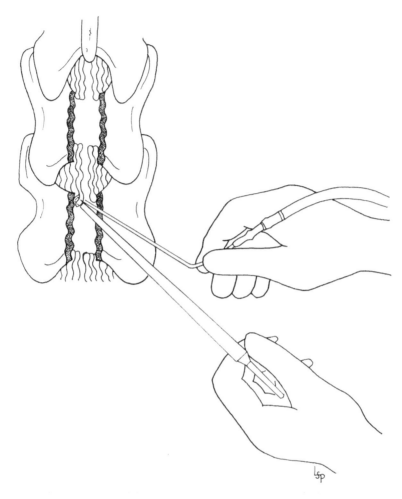

Fig. 6.15 Removal of ligamentum flavum by advancing along lateral attachment from either edge and peeling it off the dural lateral to medial.

6. For cross-cutting decompression of contralateral side (non-operated): removal
of most ventral portion of interspinous
ligament and visualization parallel
under lamina allowing removal of
hypertrophic ligamentum and medial
facet. (Note: Visual facilitation by tilting
table away from surgeon.)

6.10 Extraforaminal Root Decompression via Parsectomy

6.10.1 Clinical Presentation

- Painful radiculopathy—discogenic and/or stenotic.

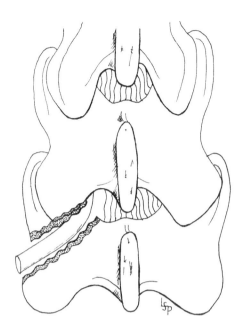

Fig. 6.16 Epidural access under upper edge of inferior lamina and completion of parsectomy.

6.10.2 Image Pathology

- Extraforaminal lateral or far-lateral herniated nucleus pulposus (HNP).
- Extraforaminal stenosis.

6.10.3 Contraindications (Relative to Significance of Potential for Instability)

- Absence of integrity of ipsilateral and/or contralateral lamina (of caudal vertebra)..
- Contralateral pars defect.

6.10.4 Operative Technique

1. Extension of unilateral exposure to lateral edge of facets.
2. Cautery clearance of pars, lateral IAP, and upper facet joint (removal of superior capsule).
3. Clear lateral upper edge of lamina with dissector.
4. Enter epidural space under superior edge of lateral lamina with 2-mm Kerrisons (▶ Fig. 6.16) (note: U-turn approach may be used to access root at foraminal entrance).
5. With sequential drilling and rongeuring, identify nerve root laterally at foraminal entrance and follow/decompress root/nerve out with parsectomy and removal of superior aspect of facets to lateral edge of joint (muscular branch of radicular artery usually cauterized).
6. Lift nerve cephalad with nerve hook and explore/locate HNP; excise and remove HNP with nerve hook and forceps with minimal interbody discectomy; explore above nerve for free disc material (▶ Fig. 6.17).

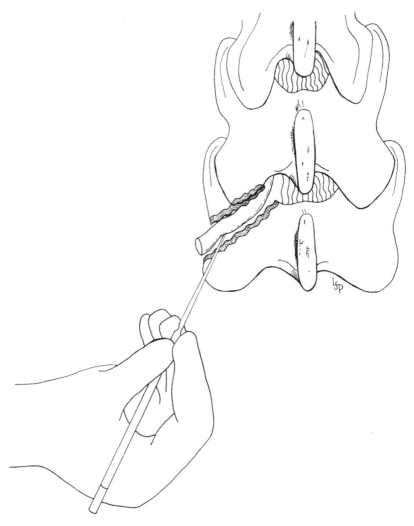

Fig. 6.17 Using nerve hook to retract and explore under nerve for disc herniation.

6.11 Extraforaminal Root Decompression with Partial Lateral Parsectomy

6.11.1 Clinical Presentation

• Painful radiculopathy—discogenic and/or stenotic.

6.11.2 Image Pathology

• Extraforaminal lateral or far-lateral HNP.
• Extraforaminal stenosis.
• Evidence of potential instability: absence of integrity of ipsilateral or contralateral lamina or of contralateral pars.

6.11.3 Contraindications

• None.

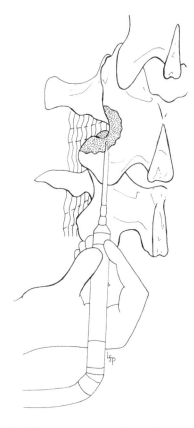

Fig. 6.18 Bony preparation for extraforaminal nerve decompression.

6.11.4 Operative Technique

1. Extension of unilateral exposure to lateral edge of facet joints.
2. Cautery clearance and then drilling/thinning of lateral IAP/pars and superior aspect of facet joint (▶ Fig. 6.18).
3. Rongeur (Kerrisons) under lateral edge of pars with separation of underlying intertransverse ligament to expose

perineural space (may require probing with nerve hook) (▶ Fig. 6.19).
4. Remove ligament with Kerrison and identify nerve and continue distal decompression with sequential removal of bone and soft tissue (muscular branch or radicular artery usually cauterized).
5. Lift nerve cephalad with nerve hook to explore/locate HNP; explore above nerve for free disc material (▶ Fig. 6.20).

6.12 Root/Dural Decompression on Operated Anatomy with Joints Intact

All decompression is done lateral to medial using bony landmarks as guide to neural elements starting at *sentinel root*.

Longitudinal decompression then proceeds along continuous bony corridor consisting of joint, pars, lamina, IAP (caudally) or joint, IAP, lamina, pars (cephalad).

- Determination of residual bony anatomy (radiographically or via records).
- Determination of sentinel root and its pedicle/overlying facet joint.
- Determination of existence of midline bony landmark (SP) to serve as guide to facet joint over sentinel root: either via SP–lamina–IAP joint or SP–lamina–pars joint.
- If midline structures (SP/lamina) are not intact, then dissect laterally to identify facet joint over sentinel root (▶ Fig. 6.21).
- Identify and clear residual IAP/lamina (cephalad) and pars/lamina (caudal).
- Remove medial aspect of superior facet/IAP/lamina with drill/rongeur to identify

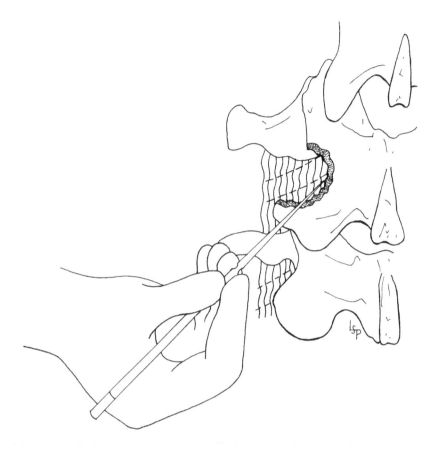

Fig. 6.19 Access to epidural space under medial edge of intertransverse ligament at pedicle.

sentinel root proximal to foramen (or inferior facet/medial pars may be removed to access root at foraminal entrance).

- Decompress sentinel root working cephalad laterally by removing medial IAP/residual lamina with detachment of cicatrix and residual ligamentum flavum from wall of canal and peeling it lateral to medial off dura; explore for discogenic compression (▶ Fig. 6.22).
- Advance cephalad along lateral corridor (IAP–lateral lamina–pars) to identify

higher joint and subsequent root/dura for similar decompression, etc., and/or advance caudally along pars–lamina–IAP to lower joint, etc. (▶ Fig. 6.23).

6.13 Multistep Process for Accurate Pedicle Screw Placement

1. Identify juncture of superior articular process (SAP) and pars at medial extension of line from midway between

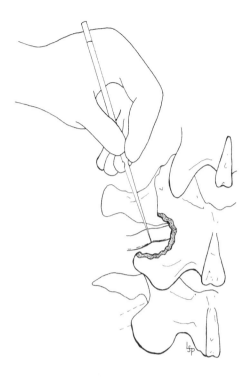

Fig. 6.20 Nerve hook retraction and exploration under nerve.

upper and lower edges of transverse process (TP).

2. Drill (matchstick) shallow transcortical defect at this site (▶ Fig. 6.24).

3. Carefully mallet marker into this defect and confirm position fluoroscopically (▶ Fig. 6.25).

4. Adjust drill hole/marker accordingly for marker to be at, or just inside, outer edge of midpedicle.

5. Confirm transcortical defect and *gently tap* down "gear-shift" probe with mallet into pedicle (under fluoroscopy); the tip will generally deflect appropriately off inner pedicle wall (resistance to gentle tapping is usually because the tip is

angled against medial wall and should be directed more laterally = raising handle for more vertical position).

6. When tip of gear-shift is seen fluoroscopically to enter the vertebral body, advance manually.

7. Measure, tap, and place appropriate screw.

6.13.1 S2 Alar Iliac Screws Placement

For the pelvic anchoring of a long lumbar or thoracolumbar fixation, an iliac connection is required. There are two common techniques used currently: iliac screws

2. Screws placed into the ilium from the second alar segment across the sacro-iliac joint.

The advantages of the latter technique (S2 alar iliac screws) are the following[1,3]:
- They do not require separate fascial incision.
- They are on the sacrum below the ilium and this low profile (especially in thinner patients) has minimal potential for painful implant prominence or tissue breakdown.
- They are in line with S1 screws and thus do not require offset connectors.
- They do not interfere with iliac graft harvest.
- They have been shown to have fewer re-operations for wound complications and instrument failure.[4]

(Note: Iliac screw placement can be done from a starting point through the inner surface of the ilium below the PSIS, which may negate some disadvantages relative to S2 alar iliac screws.)

The technique of placement:
- Starting point at lateral sacral crest at midpoint between the first and second sacral foramen (▶ Fig. 6.26).
- Laterally angled (in axial plane) at 40–50 degrees and sagittally angled at about 85 degrees *relative to posterior surface of sacrum* (i.e., angled upward with slight convergence on a line parallel to end plate of S1) (▶ Fig. 6.27).

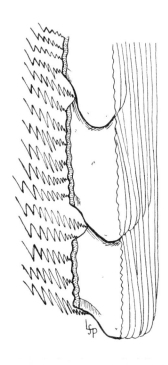

Fig. 6.21 Direct exposure of facet (right side) for access to sentinel root.

placed solely within the ilium proper from a point just anterior to the posterior superior iliac spine (PSIS).

1. Iliac screws placed solely within the ilium proper from a point just anterior to the posterior superior iliac spine (PSIS).

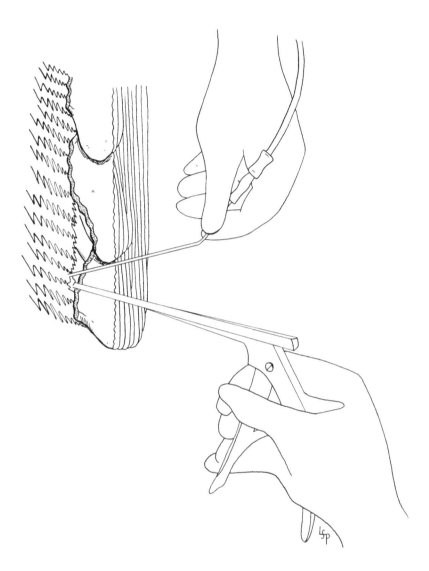

Fig. 6.22 Advancing laterally along root/dural for removal of medial facet, residual ligamentum flavum, and cicatrix, peeling lateral to medial.

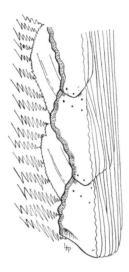

Fig. 6.23 Advancing along lateral corridor for access to next root.

The margin of safety in the axial plane is 15 degrees (i.e., angled laterally no less than 25 degrees) and about 10 degrees sagittally (i.e., representing any divergence with a line parallel to the sacral end plate).

(Note: The sagittal angle is commonly described as being 40 degrees caudally but this is relative to the operating room floor and does not take into account variability in patient position and pelvic incidence).

- The trajectory on fluoroscopic guidance is the anterior inferior iliac spine or slightly lower to the notch that it makes with the acetabulum (anteroposterior and lateral fluoroscopic views showing the sciatic notch is recommended) (▶ Fig. 6.28).
- Development of the hole can be with 2.5-mm drill through SI joint and then 3.2-mm drill.
- A thin and pointed "gear-shift" probe also can be gently malleted along the proper projection, which allows for easy adjustment under fluoroscopic guidance.
- A "tear-drop" view of ilium will confirm proper position within.

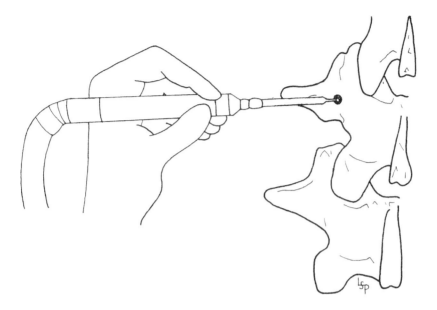

Fig. 6.24 Matchstick drilling to make shallow transcortical depression for placement of marker.

- Polyaxial screws of 80 to 100 mm in length and 8 to 10 mm in diameter.

6.14 Repair and Wound Closure after Incidental Durotomy

1. Use only small (#7) multiperforated suction to avoid rootlet aspiration injury.

2. If root/filament herniation through defect occurs, gently push it back into dura with closed bayonet forceps and hold in with paddy as aspirating cerebrospinal fluid (CSF). (Note: if root herniates out in strangulating fashion and cannot be reduced, then emergent removal of more bone is necessary to allow extension of durotomy or large separate adjacent dural opening for fast removal of CSF.)

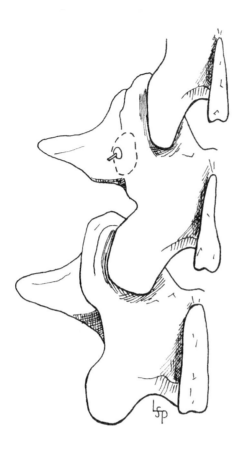

Fig. 6.25 Marker in place for fluoroscopic verification of pedicle entry.

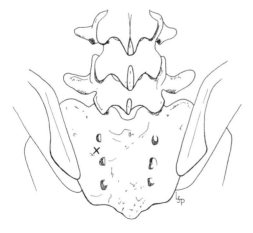

Fig. 6.26 Starting point for S2 alar iliac screws between S1 and S2 foramen.

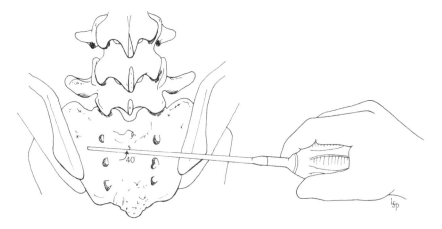

Fig. 6.27 Projection of drill or probe as referenced to sacral surface 40-50 degrees elevated in axial plane and 5 degrees cephalad in the sagittal plane (slightly convergent to sacral end plate).

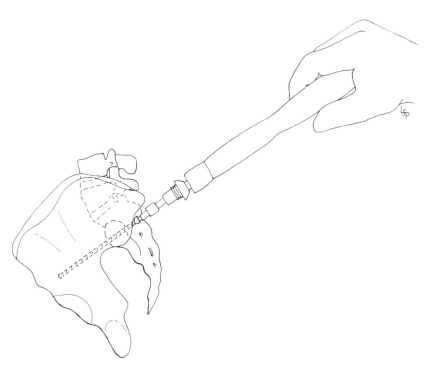

Fig. 6.28 Sagittal trajectory to AIIS or lower notch as visualized on lateral fluoroscopy.

3. After sufficient CSF removal, nerve elements will retract into dura.
4. Best water-tight closure of dura done with one free-end knot by double running (shoe string) (▶ Fig. 6.29).
5. Coverage of closed durotomy with tissue glue optional.
6. Water-tight closure of fascia with large (#1) running locked, nonabsorbable suture reinforced with large (#1) interrupted absorbable sutures (▶ Fig. 6.30).
7. Accurate skin approximation using superficial subcutaneous sutures and running locked suture on skin.

(Note: Steps #5–7 dependent on surgeon's confidence in water-tight dural closure.)

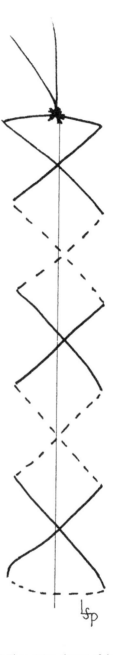

Fig. 6.29 Shoe string closure of dura—one free-end knot.

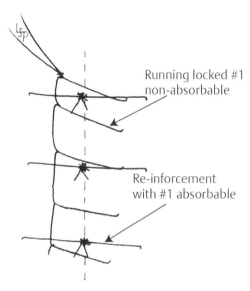

Fig. 6.30 Water-tight reinforced closure of deep fascia.

Running locked #1 non-absorbable

Re-inforcement with #1 absorbable

References

[1] Chang HS, Fujisawa N, Tsuchiya T, Oya S, Matsui T. Degenerative spondylolisthesis does not affect the outcome of unilateral laminotomy with bilateral decompression in patients with lumbar stenosis. Spine. 2014; 39(5):400–408

[2] Kebaish KM. Sacropelvic fixation: techniques and complications. Spine. 2010; 35(25):2245–2251

[3] Lee S-H, Jin W, Kim K-T, Suk K-S, Lee J-H, Seo G-W. Trajectory of transsacral iliac screw for lumbo-pelvic fixation: a 3-dimensional computed tomography study. J Spinal Disord Tech. 2011; 24 (3):151–156

[4] Mazur MD, Ravindra VM, Schmidt MH, et al. Unplanned reoperation after lumbopelvic fixation with S-2 alar-iliac screws or iliac bolts. J Neurosurg Spine. 2015; 23(1):67–76

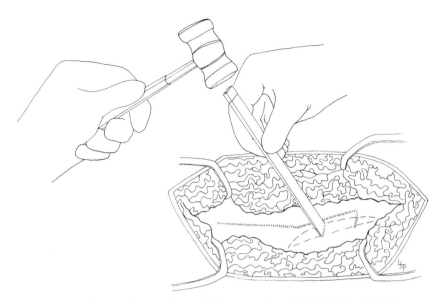

Fig. 7.7 Transverse transcortical incisions of ilium with osteotomes after fascial incisions.

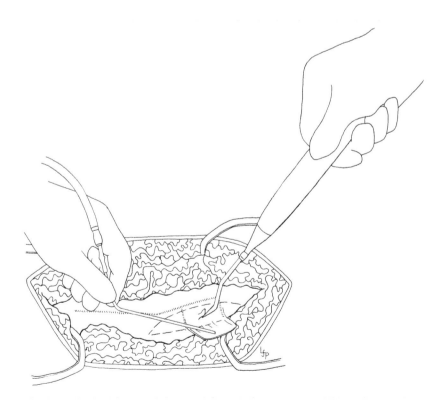

Fig. 7.8 Cortical flap of the ilium hinged laterally with the medial leaf of the fascia preserved.

References

[1] Wiltse LL. The paraspinal sacrospinalis-splitting approach to the lumbar spine. Clin Orthop Relat Res. 1973(91):48–57

[2] Weaver EN, Jr. Lateral intramuscular planar approach to the lumbar spine and sacrum. Technical note. J Neurosurg Spine. 2007; 7(2):270–273

8 Minimally Invasive Surgical Method

James B. Macon

Abstract

Minimally invasive surgery (MIS), as applied to the lumbar spine, includes many techniques for both decompression and fusion as alternatives to the open spine procedures described elsewhere in this text. Although decompression can be performed with smaller access than fusion, MIS means the minimal access that can safely accomplish the individual surgical goal. Each MIS approach is designed to reduce unnecessary tissue trauma and thereby reduce postoperative pain, blood loss, infection rate and length of stay relative to the open surgery counterparts and thereby optimize value for patients. This chapter provides in some detail a step-by-step guide for performance of some commonly employed approaches for MIS decompression for lumbar disc herniations and spinal stenosis as well as three approaches to perform MIS fusion for lumbar segmental instability including TLIF, PLIF and XLIF. The risks and benefits of each procedure are described as they should be presented to patients prior to surgery by the operating surgeon. The relative benefits of lumbar MIS versus open techniques are discussed as well as the opportunities for future advancement of the MIS method.

Keywords: MIS, minimally invasive lumbar decompression, fusion, discectomy, herniation, stenosis, foraminotomy, laminectomy, TLIF, PLIF, XLIF

Everything should be made as simple as possible, but not simpler.

Albert Einstein

8.1 Introduction

The concept of minimally invasive surgery (MIS) originated in the 1980s, but its application to the lumbar spine has been credited to the 1997 publication by Foley and Smith,[1] who introduced the minimally invasive endoscopic lumbar microdiscectomy. MIS is defined as the minimal access that allows accomplishment of the surgical goal. MIS is not defined by incision size since that will vary depending on the type of procedure performed (i.e., discectomy or fusion). The minimally invasive discectomy involves inserting a tubular port directly through the paraspinal muscles by splitting the muscles using concentric dilators, then passing the working port over the final dilator. This muscle-splitting approach of Wiltse[2] minimizes muscle trauma and pain without damaging subsequent muscle function.[3] The tube trajectory is monitored and adjusted using biplane fluoroscopy in order that placement will be required only once and be precisely where the surgical pathology is accessible. Multiple attempts to place the tube must be avoided to prevent unnecessary muscle trauma.

This "simple" method allows the surgery to be performed through the smallest access that will allow the procedure to be accomplished safely and successfully.[4] The goal of the MIS approach is to minimize tissue trauma, thereby reducing postoperative pain, blood loss, infection rates, operative time, and hospital length of stay. All of these advantages would appear to be cost-effective in favor of the MIS approach. The disadvantage and constraint of working the limited space at the bottom of the tube has been countered by introducing fiberoptic light sources from the endoscope and using bayonet-handled instruments that do not impair the line of sight when looking down the tube. Now the operating microscope, that is ubiquitous in the neurosurgical operating suite, is used instead of the endoscope to preserve binocular vision and depth perception. The parameters that define the transtubular approach must be optimized including tube length and diameter with each procedure in order that the surgical goal can be accomplished successfully. Naturally a tube that is too small or positioned with the wrong trajectory will not allow a successful procedure. Attempting to perform surgery through too narrow a tube preventing adequate visualization or placement of instruments is dangerous and would be an example of "simpler than possible." There is a balancing act between minimally invasive access and safety that will be determined by each spine surgeon based on individual patience and skill with the goal of providing the best outcome for patients. Attempting to reduce the exposure to a size that is too small to safely achieve the surgical goal with an optimal outcome would be "simpler than possible" and should be avoided by all MIS spine surgeons. However, the safe exposure size needed to accomplish the surgical goals will vary with the patience, skill, training, and experience of each surgeon.

When performed properly, this method is brilliant in its simplicity and as a consequence increases value for patients. In order to perform MIS surgery, there are many new factors and technical details that must be considered and consequently only surgeons well trained in open procedures should attempt the MIS approach. Although the procedure is conceptually simple, it is technically different from the open technique. **It is important to stress that experience with open surgery is essential before attempting the MIS approach**.

When it comes to comparing MIS relative to open surgery, it is accurate to say that "less is more" when lumbar MIS procedures are performed correctly and safely and all the surgical goals are accomplished. Comparison studies have shown that MIS techniques have results and complication rates comparable to open procedures.[5] Considering the added advantages of less surgical tissue trauma, the MIS method

optimizes value for patients and at the same time may prove to be cost-effective. The following descriptions of MIS are intended for comparison with the previously described open surgeries in prior chapters of this text.

8.2 Surgical Decision: Open or MIS of the Lumbar Spine

8.2.1 Patient–Surgeon Interaction in Surgical Decision-Making

- When the decision has been made by the surgeon and patient that surgery is indicated, the patient must be informed of the alternatives available for treatment.
- The risks and possible complications of the open versus MIS methods should be explained in detail.
- Together the patient and surgeon should choose the procedure that is most likely to safely provide the optimal outcome.
- To avoid unnecessary surgery, the pathology seen on imaging must adequately account for the patient's clinical presentation.

8.2.2 Operative Plan for MIS the Approach

- The choice of procedure will provide direct minimally invasive access to the symptomatic pathology with no unnecessary components to avoid collateral damage (i.e., no fusion without instability on imaging and no extra levels without indication).
- Procedures designed for treatment of pain alone will only be performed if the pain generator has been confidently identified with preoperative objective radicular neurological deficits, relief with nerve root blocks, or provocative and

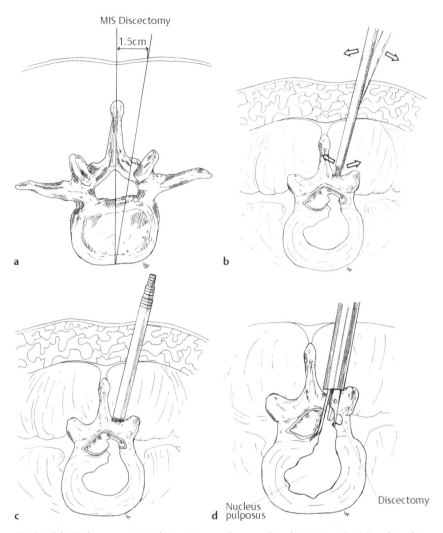

Fig. 8.1 (a) MIS decompression tube trajectory and paramedian skin incision site 1.5 cm lateral to midline. **(b)** Placement of initial inner dilator for tube placement trajectory confirmation and wanding to prepare lamina for working tube contact. **(c)** Placement of dilators in preparation for insertion of the working tube. **(d)** Removal of herniated disc with nerve root retractor protecting the dura.

- The operating microscope will then be positioned to allow illumination and visualization of the operative site at the bottom of the tube. The operating microscope must be moved out of the field in order to rotate the C-arm into position from this point forward in the

procedure. There will usually be soft tissue consisting of muscle and ligament obscuring the bone surface. After palpation with instruments (Penfield 4), the soft tissue is removed with monopolar cautery to expose and allow identification of the bony margins of the lamina and facet. (Only bipolar cautery is used for the remainder of the procedure.) If the expected appearance of the bone is not what is seen, repeat biplane fluoroscopy as necessary to determine if the trajectory requires adjustment. This can be performed by loosening the flex arm and tilting the tube ("wanding") in the required direction.

- The laminotomy, foraminotomy, and discectomy are then performed through the access tube using bayonet-angled instruments in a manner identical to the open surgery (▶ Fig. 8.1d). The illumination and visualization obtained with the operating microscope is superior to loupes or an endoscope. A two-level unilateral decompression can be performed through a single approach by making the incision midway between the two disc spaces and wanding the tube to each level with final position determined by fluoroscopy (▶ Fig. 8.2a).
- After the decompression is complete, the working tube is removed, hemostasis achieved, and sutures are placed in the fascia and subcutaneous and subcuticular tissues, followed by a small dressing.

Complications of Minimally Invasive Surgery Decompression

The complications of MIS decompression[7] surgery are similar to those encountered during open surgery, including infection, bleeding, dural tear with cerebrospinal fluid (CSF) leak, and nerve root injury. There are certain issues specific to the MIS decompression technique that must be considered to prevent complications.

- Bleeding must be meticulously controlled as encountered in order to allow visualization in the working tube. Since bleeding must be controlled at each step to perform the operation, significant postoperative hematomas are very rare.
- Infection prophylaxis with broad spectrum perioperative antibiotics combined with meticulous sterile technique will reduce the incidence of infection to a minimum. Infection rates should be less than 1%.[8]
- During discectomy or foraminotomy, when operating around the thecal sac, the dura must be retracted with a right-angled suction retractor since conventional retractors will block visualization, especially when there is significant epidural bleeding. If a dural tear occurs, the narrow tube diameter makes conventional primary suture of the dura technically difficult requiring microvascular clips, so the repair method usually consists of application of a synthetic collagen or fascial patch covered by fibrin sealant and reinforced by muscle or fat. A significant or persistent CSF leak will require a lumbar subarachnoid drain for CSF diversion. Failure to adequately stop a CSF leak should not be ignored since the leak increases the risk of infection and meningitis. A persistent leak may require a direct suture repair via conversion to open technique or another open surgery. Dural tear risk is 2 to 10% depending on the surgeon's experience and skill.
- The risk of dural tear is significant during the dilation process that requires docking the guidewire under biplane fluoroscopy (AP and lateral), then passing small-diameter inner dilators blindly over the guidewire. It is essential to monitor this process with lateral fluoroscopy so the guidewire does not bind to the inner dilator and get pushed blindly through the interlaminar space, puncturing the dura and potentially injuring one or more nerve roots.
- Wrong side surgery is possible with MIS decompressions. Be certain to verify the side to be operated on by checking the preoperative imaging study before the skin incision is made. Wrong level surgery is no more likely than open surgery as long as the level is confirmed with intraoperative fluoroscopy (or computed tomography [CT]).

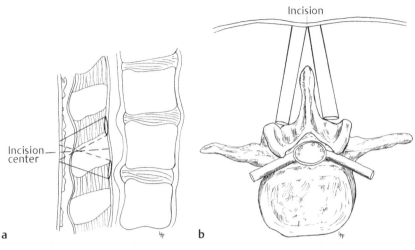

Fig. 8.2 **(a)** Two adjacent level ipsilateral decompression tubular approaches. **(b)** Same level bilateral decompression tubular approach angles.

8.4.2 Bilateral Decompression (MIS Dual-Tube Medial Foraminotomy)

Clinical Presentation

- Painful bilateral lower extremity radiculopathy.
- One-level bilateral pain generator.

Image Pathology

- Bilateral medial foraminal stenosis due to disc protrusion or facet hypertrophy.
- Bilateral subarticular (lateral recess) stenosis with nerve root compression.
- Bilateral disc protrusions with nerve root compression in the lateral recess.

Contraindications (Relative)

- Large central disc herniation.
- Far lateral or extraforaminal disc herniation.
- Central canal stenosis due to facet/ligament hypertrophy.
- Lumbar spondylolisthesis.

Operative Technique

The operative technique (▶ Fig. 8.2b) is midline incision (20–24 mm length) and two fascial incisions (1 cm lateral to spinous process) with tubular diameter (18–22 mm).

- After induction of general endotracheal anesthesia, the patient is placed prone on a spinal frame and the back prepped and draped in the standard manner. The incision size should be 2 mm greater than the anticipated working tube diameter to prevent skin necrosis due to stretch. Be certain to verify the side and level to be operated on by checking the preoperative imaging study before the skin incision is made.
- Place a 22-gauge spinal needle in the midline at the center of the anticipated incision site to the depth of the lamina. The needle is directed from the midline laterally 20 to 30 degrees passing paramedian 1 to 2 cm lateral to the spinous process toward the medial facet and lateral lamina (▶ Fig. 8.2b). Note the level of needle insertion to assure it correlates with the imaging and pathological

condition in the lateral spinal canal. Use biplane fluoroscopy to accurately determine the required tube length and trajectory. Measure the final depth of the needle to confirm the tube length.

- Make the skin incision (20–24 mm) only after absolute certainty that the proper level, trajectory, and position with respect to the surgical pathology have been determined.
- A fascial incision (20–24 mm) is made 1 cm lateral to the edge of the spinous process. Pass the guidewire through the fascial incision to the level of the facet and dock in bone, making certain that the docking site is not too near the interlaminar space, and confirm its position with biplane fluoroscopy. Pass the inner dilator over the guidewire rotating the dilator until it hits the facet. Then again confirm that the guidewire and dilator are properly positioned using biplane fluoroscopy before proceeding with dilation. Pass additional dilators until the desired working diameter (18–22 mm, depending on the pathology) is achieved.
- Pass the working tube over the dilators. Remove the guidewire and dilators keeping the working tube steady to prevent migration and secure to the flex arm attached to the operating table. Do not release the working channel until a firm attachment is secured. The working tube must be firmly compressed against the lamina and facet and secured to prevent posterior movement of the tube that allows the muscle to creep into the work space. Final confirmation of the tube position is then made with biplane fluoroscopy before beginning any surgery. Since localization is not dependent on visualization of anatomical structures, accurate radiological localization is essential.
- The operating microscope will then be positioned to allow illumination and visualization of the operative site at the bottom of the tube. The surgeon will stand on the contralateral side to the

pathology. The operating microscope must be moved out of the field in order to rotate the C-arm into position from this point forward in the procedure. There will be soft tissue consisting of muscle and ligament obscuring the bone surface. After palpation with instruments (Penfield 4), the soft tissue is removed with monopolar cautery to expose and allow identification of the bony margins of the lamina and facet. (Only bipolar cautery is used for the remainder of the procedure.) If the expected appearance of the bone is not what is seen, repeat biplane fluoroscopy is necessary to determine if the trajectory requires adjustment. This can be performed by loosening the flex arm and tilting the tube ("wanding") in the required direction.

- The lateral laminectomy and medial foraminotomy are then performed through the access tube using bayonet-angled instruments in a manner identical to the unilateral decompression. The main difference is that the tube is angled about 10 degrees laterally (▶ Fig. 8.2b). The illumination and visualization obtained with the operating microscope is superior to loupes or endoscope. After the pathology is removed on one side, the tube is removed, hemostasis achieved, and sutures are placed in the fascia; then, attention is turned to the contralateral side.
- Once the decompression is completed on one side working from the opposite side of the operating table, repeat the process to decompress the contralateral lateral recess and medial foramen to accomplish the bilateral decompression as necessary (▶ Fig. 8.2b).
- After the second decompression, the tube is removed, hemostasis is achieved, and sutures are placed in the fascia and subcutaneous and subcuticular tissues, followed by a small dressing.
- The advantage of this approach is that bilateral decompressions can be

performed through a single midline vertical skin incision without disrupting the stabilizing midline spinous processes or ligaments constituting the posterior lumbar tension band. This method is only to be used when there is no significant central stenosis or pre-existing instability.

Complications

- Bleeding.
- Infection.
- Nerve root injury.
- Dural tear with CSF leak.
- Instability due to excessive bilateral facetectomy.

8.4.3 Laminectomy (MIS Unilateral Single-Tube Bilateral Decompression)

Clinical Presentation

- Neurogenic claudication (bilateral).
- Single-level stenotic radiculopathy.
- Central stenosis and bilateral foraminal or lateral recess stenosis.

Image Pathology

- Single-level severe/moderate central stenosis with significant ligamentum flavum hypertrophy.
- Bilateral focal (< 2 cm length) lateral recess and central canal stenosis.

Contraindications

- Large central disc herniation with cauda equina decompression.

Operative Technique

The operative technique (▶ Fig. 8.3)[9,10,11,12,13] is paramedian incision (between 1.5 and 3 cm lateral to midline) with tubular diameter (22 mm).

Ipsilateral nerve root decompression is performed via a more lateral trajectory (1) and tube placement (as previously described for unilateral decompression) with modifications as detailed below. Contralateral decompression is performed via the more medial trajectory (2) as described below (▶ Fig. 8.3a).

1. After induction of general endotracheal anesthesia, the patient is placed prone on a spinal frame and the back prepped and draped in the standard manner. The incision size should be 2 mm greater than the anticipated working tube diameter. Be certain to verify the side and level to be operated on by checking the preoperative imaging study before the skin incision is made.

2. Place a 22-gauge spinal needle in the center of the anticipated skin incision site 2.5 cm lateral to the midline (▶ Fig. 8.3a) to the depth of the ipsilateral lamina. Note the level of needle insertion to assure it correlates with the imaging and pathological condition. Use biplane fluoroscopy to accurately determine the required tube length and trajectory. Measure the final depth of the needle to confirm the tube length.

3. Make the skin incision (24 mm) only after absolute certainty that the proper level, trajectory, and position with respect to the surgical pathology have been determined. After the skin incision, retract subcutaneous tissues to the fascial level and sharply open horizontally to allow required medial to lateral tube trajectory adjustments.

4. Place the guidewire through the fascial incision to the level of the facet and dock on bone, making certain that the docking site is not too near the interlaminar space, and confirm its position with biplane fluoroscopy. Pass the inner dilator over the guidewire rotating the dilator until it hits the facet. Then again confirm that the guidewire and dilator are properly positioned using biplane fluoroscopy before

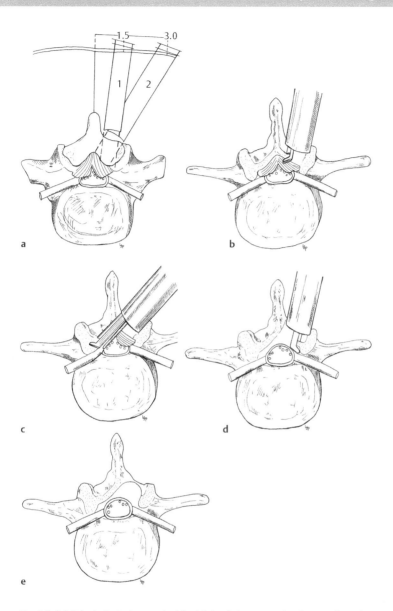

Fig. 8.3 (a) Tube trajectories required for bilateral decompression from unilateral approach: ipsilateral (1) and contralateral (2). **(b)** Step 1 ipsilateral laminotomy with preservation of ligamentum flavum. **(c)** Step 2 contralateral decompression with medial facetectomy using the rongeur with adjacent retractor protecting the dura. **(d)** Step 3 ipsilateral decompression after resection of ligament and medial facetectomy with the rongeur. **(e)** Step 4 completed bilateral decompression from a unilateral approach.

proceeding with dilation. Pass additional dilators until the desired working diameter (18–22 mm, depending on the pathology) is achieved.

5. Pass the working tube over the dilators. Remove the guidewire and dilators keeping the working tube steady to prevent migration and secure to the flex arm attached to the operating table. Do not release the working channel until a firm attachment is secured. The working tube must be firmly compressed against the lamina and facet and secured to prevent posterior movement of the tube that allows the muscle to creep into the work space. Final confirmation of the tube position is then made with biplane fluoroscopy before beginning any surgery. Since localization is not dependent on visualization of anatomical structures, accurate radiological localization is essential.

6. The operating microscope will then be positioned to allow illumination and visualization of the operative site at the bottom of the tube. The operating microscope must be moved out of the field in order to rotate the C-arm into position from this point forward in the procedure. There will be soft tissue consisting of muscle and ligament obscuring the bone surface. After palpation with instruments (Penfield 4), the soft tissue is removed with monopolar cautery to expose and allow identification of the bony margins of the lamina and facet. (Only bipolar cautery is used for the remainder of the procedure.) If the expected appearance of the bone is not what is seen, repeat biplane fluoroscopy is necessary to determine if the trajectory requires adjustment. This can be performed by loosening the flex arm and tilting the tube ("wanding") in the required direction.

7. Initial ipsilateral exposure (step 1) is performed with the tube at the skin level positioned 1 cm from the midline (trajectory 1) by separating the ligamentum flavum from the lamina with a curved curette and then performing a laminectomy with the drill and Kerrison rongeurs to the cranial margin of the ligament wide enough to decompress the stenotic spinal canal. The ligament is left in place to protect the dura during the contralateral decompression (▸ Fig. 8.3b).

8. Then the tube is released and wanded medially with the tube at the skin level 3 cm lateral to the midline to expose the base of the spinous process and achieve the exposure (trajectory 2) required for the contralateral decompression (▸ Fig. 8.3c). The tube is then secured to the operating table with the flex arm. The table is turned away from the surgeon to allow a direct approach to the contralateral lamina (step 2). The Kerrison rongeur and high-speed drill are then used to remove the base of the spinous process and resect the inner cortex of the contralateral lamina (▸ Fig. 8.3c). The dura is protected by leaving the ligament intact and gently retracting with a multiperforated no. 7 suction tube during the drilling. Bleeding is controlled with bone wax applied on the back of a Penfield no. 4 instrument. The laminar resection is continued until the contralateral facet is encountered. Care is taken to preserve the outer cortex of the lamina to insure stability of the spinous process. It is essential to control bone bleeding from the residual laminar and facet surface with bone wax to prevent postoperative hematoma.

9. The contralateral decompression is completed by drilling the medial facet and performing a contralateral foraminotomy with a 40-degree angled 2-mm Kerrison rongeur (▸ Fig. 8.3c). After all drilling is completed, the contralateral ligamentum flavum is removed to expose the dura and a ball tip probe is utilized to confirm

adequate decompression of the nerve roots of the cauda equina. After completion of the contralateral decompression, the tube is removed to the original position for completion of the ipsilateral decompression (step 3).

10. The ipsilateral laminectomy, foraminotomy, and discectomy are then performed through the access tube using bayonet- or right-angled instruments in a manner identical to unilateral decompression surgery. The residual ligament is removed to expose the dura and then a medial facetectomy and foraminotomy are performed with the Kerrison rongeur (▶ Fig. 8.3d). If discectomy is required for central canal decompression, it is performed from the ipsilateral approach. The adequacy of the bilateral decompression is checked with a ball-tipped probe or angled flat dural separator (▶ Fig. 8.3e). The illumination and visualization obtained with the operating microscope is superior to loupes or endoscope especially for the contralateral decompression.

11. After the ipsilateral pathology is resected and the decompression completed, the working tube is removed (▶ Fig. 8.3e), hemostasis achieved, and the sutures are placed in the fascial incisions and subcutaneous and subcuticular tissues; then, a small dressing is applied.

12. The advantage of this procedure is the reduction of risk of iatrogenic instability by preserving the midline tension band composed of the spinous process and midline ligaments and minimizing the extent of facetectomy especially on the contralateral side. This method has been proposed as superior to open decompression and fusion for stable grade I or II spondylolisthesis with no motion on pre-op flexion–extension X-rays, thereby avoiding the risks of fixation and fusion.[14]

Complications

- Bleeding from drilled contralateral lamina.
- Infection.
- Dural tear with CSF leak.
- Residual contralateral stenosis.
- Cauda equina compression due to retraction or hematoma.

8.4.4 Far Lateral Nerve Root Decompression (MIS Lateral Discectomy)

Clinical Presentation

- Painful single-level radiculopathy: discogenic and/or stenotic.

Image Pathology

- Lateral foraminal or extraforaminal far-lateral HNP (herniated nucleus pulposus) best seen on magnetic resonance (MR) scan (▶ Fig. 8.4a).
- Lateral foraminal stenosis best seen on CT scan.

Contraindications

- Medial foraminal or lateral recess disc herniations.

Operative Technique

The operative technique (▶ Fig. 8.4)[15,16,17] is paramedian incision (~4–5 cm lateral to the midline) with tubular diameter (18–22 mm).

- After induction of general endotracheal anesthesia, the patient is placed prone on a spinal frame and the back prepped and draped in the standard manner. The C-arm fluoroscope should be draped into the operative field. The incision size should be 2 mm greater than the anticipated working tube diameter. Be certain to verify the side to be operated on by checking the

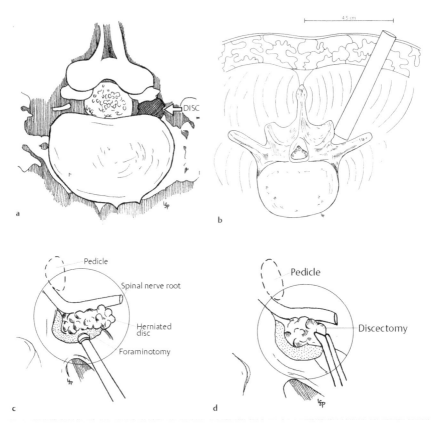

Fig. 8.4 **(a)** Axial scan demonstrates nerve root compression at the level of a lateral foraminal disc herniation (open arrow). **(b)** MIS decompression tube positioned for lateral discectomy with proper trajectory passing through a paramedian skin incision centered 4.5 cm lateral to the midline. **(c)** View through MIS decompression tube with drill performing lateral foraminotomy to expose the nerve root compressed in the foramen by a lateral disc herniation. **(d)** Lateral discectomy performed through the MIS decompression tube.

preoperative imaging study before the skin incision is made.

- Place a 22-gauge spinal needle in the center of the anticipated incision site to the depth of the lateral facet. Note the disc level of needle insertion to assure it correlates with the imaging and pathological condition. Use biplane fluoroscopy to accurately determine the required tube length and trajectory of the working tube. Measure the final depth of the needle to confirm the tube length.

- Make the skin incision (20–24 mm) only after absolute certainty that the proper level, trajectory, and position with respect to the surgical pathology have been determined.
- Place the guidewire to the level of the lateral facet and dock in bone, making certain that the docking site is not too near the foramen to avoid the exiting nerve root, and confirm its position with biplane fluoroscopy. Pass the inner dilator over the guidewire rotating the dilator until it hits the lateral facet. Then

again confirm that the guidewire and dilator are properly positioned using biplane fluoroscopy before proceeding with dilation. Then remove the guidewire. Pass additional dilators over the inner dilator until the desired working tube diameter (18–22 mm, depending on the pathology) is achieved. The working tube is secured to the operating table with a flex arm being careful to keep the desired depth and trajectory (▶ Fig. 8.4b).

• The operating microscope will then be positioned to allow illumination and visualization of the operative site at the bottom of the tube. At this point, the intertransverse ligament and fascia must be opened to allow exposure of the exiting nerve root passing beneath the pedicle (▶ Fig. 8.4c). Then working medial and caudal to the exiting nerve root, the herniated disc and disc space will be identified in Kambin's triangle.[18] The remainder of the procedure is done as described for the open technique: open the lateral foramen, remove the disc, and decompress the exiting nerve root and sensory ganglion (▶ Fig. 8.4d). Placement of a local anesthetic and steroid-soaked fat graft over the ganglion prior to closing will reduce postoperative radicular pain due to radiculitis. A fusion is not needed if the medial facet joint is left intact.

• After the pathology is resected, the working tube is removed, hemostasis achieved, and then sutures are placed in the fascia and subcutaneous and subcuticular tissues, followed by a small dressing.

Complications

• Bleeding.
• Infection.
• Dural tear with nerve root injury or CSF leak.
• Wrong side surgery.
• Chronic radiculitis.

8.4.5 Laminectomy (MIS Midline Approach for Bilateral Laminectomy)

Introduction

The MIS approach to complete laminectomy for extensive circumferential canal stenosis (>2 cm) with cauda equina compression requires a larger exposure than for decompression of a single nerve root. The tube must expand in the muscle to allow multilevel exposure of up to two laminae. Some have claimed that the need for expandable tubes means the approach is no longer MIS, but "mini-open." However, the described MIS approach below provides the minimal exposure to accomplish the surgical goal of complete decompression of the cauda equina and thereby qualifies as MIS. The laminectomy is performed by the piecemeal removal of bone rather than the "en bloc" approach due to the difficulty removing large specimens through the tube although a hemilamina may be removed "en bloc" if preferred. Due to the wide exposure obtained, a posterolateral fusion may be performed if desired with or without percutaneous pedicle screw fixation.

Clinical Presentation

• Neurogenic claudication (bilateral).
• Multilevel stenotic radiculopathy.

Image Pathology

• Single- or two-level severe/moderate central stenosis with significant ligamentum flavum and facet hypertrophy (>2 cm length).
• Bilateral lateral recess and central canal stenosis.
• Large central disc herniation with cauda equina decompression.

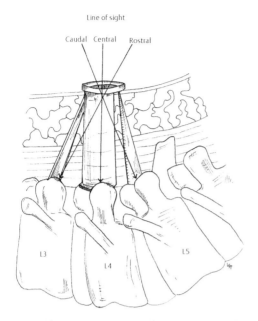

Line of sight

Caudal Central   Rostral

L3

L4

L5

Fig. 8.5 Placement of a midline expandable tube for two-level complete laminectomy through a midline vertical skin incision of 34 mm length. Changing the line of sight through the operating microscope allows increased visualization (2–3X varying with tube length) at the base of the expanded conical tube despite the small incision size.

Contraindications

- High-grade spondylolisthesis (> 1) with instability requiring reduction or multi-level fusion.

Operative Technique

The operative technique (▶ Fig. 8.5) is midline incision of 30 to 36 mm length and tubular size (28–34 mm).

- After induction of general endotracheal anesthesia, the patient is placed prone on a spinal frame and the back prepped and draped in the standard manner. The midline incision size should be 2 mm greater than the anticipated working tube diameter.
- Place a 22-gauge spinal needle in the center of the anticipated incision sites to the depth of the lamina. Note the level of needle insertion to assure it correlates with the imaging and pathological condition. Use biplane fluoroscopy to accurately determine the required tube length and trajectory. Measure the final depth of the needle to confirm the tube length.

- Make the skin incision (30–36 mm) only after absolute certainty that the proper level, trajectory, and position with respect to the surgical pathology have been determined. Dissect to the level of the midline fascia and place a self-retaining retractor. Dissect the spinous processes at the levels to be decompressed with cutting cautery and a Cobb periosteal elevator. Remove the spinous processes and ligaments with a Leksell rongeur. Place the expandable working tube without dilation to the level of the lamina and secure the tube with a flexible arm to the operating table. Then expand the working to in a rostral–caudal direction to expose to levels for the two-level complete laminectomy. The operating microscope will then be positioned to allow illumination and visualization of the operative site at the bottom of the tube. By adjusting the line of sight of the operating microscope through the tube, full expansion of the conical tube will allow visualization of the laminae two to three times greater than the incision size varying with the tube length (▶ Fig. 8.5).

- Perform the laminectomy after thinning the lamina with a 3-mm cutting burr with 2- and 3-mm Kerrison rongeurs. Then resect the ligamentum flavum to expose the lumbar dura. Extend the laminectomy laterally to the medial pedicle and perform medial facetectomy and foraminotomy until all exiting nerve roots are decompressed. If there is a midline disc herniation, it may be removed by approaching the disc from each side while gently retracting the dura containing the nerve roots of the cauda equina, but never more than 50% of the thecal sac diameter to prevent nerve root stretch injury that may cause cauda equina syndrome.
- When the decompression is completed and the working tube removed, an epidural drain may be placed if hemostasis is questionable and led out through a separate incision directed rostrally.
- The fascia is closed with interrupted resorbable sutures, then subcutaneous tissue, followed by subcuticular skin sutures and a small dressing.

Complications

- Bleeding and epidural hematoma.
- Infection.
- Dural tear with CSF leak.
- Instability due to bilateral facetectomy and resection of midline tension band.

8.5 Minimally Invasive Surgery Fusion Techniques

8.5.1 Transforaminal Lumbar Interbody Fusion

Introduction

The MIS approach to spinal fusion requires a larger exposure than the decompression surgery. The tubes placed for pedicle screw fixation (currently the standard of care for spinal fusion due to high fixation rates) must expand in the muscle to allow pedicle-to-pedicle exposure. Some have claimed that the need for expandable tubes means the approach is no longer MIS, but "mini-open." [19,20] However, even considering the expansion, the MIS transforaminal lumbar interbody fusion (TLIF) as described is less invasive than methods requiring four to six incisions of 2 cm length to allow "percutaneous" pedicle screw fixation.[21,22] As previously stated, Wiltse and others have described a paraspinal approach to the lumbar spine. The MIS approach for lumbar fusion uses the same concept, but not the natural planes between muscles to approach the spine. Instead the transtubular approach uses a muscle-splitting technique directly through the muscle using the shortest route to the pathology that causes little more trauma to muscles than retraction in the natural anatomical planes. This is because the working tube is a less traumatic device by virtue of its smaller diameter (just wide enough for pedicle-to-pedicle exposure) and smoother surface than those larger retractors used to keep the natural muscle planes open.

A variety of approach angles have been developed for MIS lumbar interbody fusion (LIF) including posterior lumbar interbody fusion (PLIF), TLIF, and direct lateral (extreme lumbar interbody fusion [XLIF] or lateral lumbar interbody fusion [LLIF]; ▶ Fig. 8.6a).[21,22] The anterior approaches to the lumbar spine, including open anterior lumbar interbody fusion (ALIF), oblique lumbar interbody fusion (OLIF), and transtubular L5–S1 AxiaLIF, directly expose the bowel, ureters, and great vessels to injury, and are not included as MIS alternatives since they are not comparable to the open procedures presented in this chapter. The choice of approach for MIS fusion requires consideration of multiple individual factors related to the patient and pathology as well as surgeon preference and experience.[23]

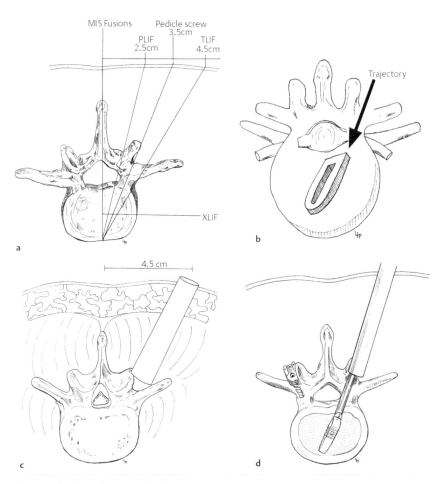

Fig. 8.6 (a) Alternative approach angles and skin incision sites for MIS lumbar interbody fusions (TLIF, PLIF, and XLIF) and pedicle screw fixation. **(b)** Trajectory for placement of TLIF interbody cage. **(c)** MIS tube placement for TLIF. **(d)** TLIF interbody cage insertion across the midline of disc space with inserter tool attached.

MIS interbody fusions require both accurate placement of interbody cages and fixation with pedicle screws and plates. Essential to the accuracy is high-quality intraoperative imaging with either C-arm fluoroscopy or O-arm CT scanning. It essential for good outcomes and patient safety that these imaging methods be employed when needed throughout the MIS fusion procedures.

Comparison of MIS fusion with open techniques confirms the advantages of minimal soft-tissue injury including less pain, fewer infections, less blood loss, faster mobilization, and shorter hospital stays.[24,25] In addition, cost-effectiveness analysis suggests lower costs with equivalent outcomes leading to higher value for patients.[26,27]

Clinical Presentation

• Painful radiculopathy affecting the exiting or traversing nerve roots at one level.

- Incapacitating antigravity axial chronic low back pain generated at one level.

Image Pathology

- Imaging evidence of excessive vertebral motion ("instability") contributory to symptomatology (or potentially so).
- Severe degenerative discogenic changes contributory to axial antigravity pain (L2–L5).

Contraindications (Relative)

- The MIS TLIF approach is applicable mainly for pathology from L2 to L5.
- Fusions of more than two levels.
- High-grade (> 1) spondylolisthesis.
- Central canal stenosis bilateral and greater than 2 cm length.

Operative Technique

The operative technique (▶ Fig. 8.6)[19,24,28] is bilateral paramedian incisions (4–5 cm laterally) of 3 to 3.6 cm length and tubular size (28–34 mm).

- After induction of general endotracheal anesthesia, the patient is placed prone on a spinal frame and the back prepped and draped in the standard manner. The bilateral incision size should be 2 mm greater than the anticipated working tube diameter.
- Place a 22-gauge spinal needle in the center of the anticipated incision sites to the depth of the lateral facet. Note the level of needle insertion to assure it correlates with the imaging and pathological condition. Use biplane fluoroscopy to accurately determine the required tube length and trajectory. Measure the final depth of the needle to confirm the tube length.
- Make the skin incision (3–3.6 cm length) only after absolute certainty that the proper level, trajectory, and position with respect to the surgical pathology have been determined 4.5 cm lateral to midline (▶ Fig. 8.6b). Dissect to the level of the fascia and open to a width 5 to 10 mm greater than the working tube diameter to accommodate pedicle-to-pedicle tube expansion.

- Place the guidewire to the level of the lateral facet and dock in bone, making certain that the docking site is not too near the foramen to avoid the exiting nerve root, and confirm its position with biplane fluoroscopy. Pass the inner dilator over the guidewire rotating the dilator until it hits the lateral facet. Then again confirm that the guidewire and dilator are properly positioned using biplane fluoroscopy before proceeding with dilation. Pass additional dilators until the desired working diameter (28–34 mm, depending on the pathology) is achieved. The working tube should be expandable (50–60 mm) beneath the fascia to allow pedicle-to-pedicle exposure (▶ Fig. 8.6c).
- The operating microscope will then be positioned to allow illumination and visualization of the operative site at the bottom of the tube. At this point, the intertransverse muscle and fascia must be opened to allow exposure of the exiting nerve root. Then working medial to the exiting nerve root, the herniated disc and disc space will be identified in Kambin's triangle (bounded by the superior aspect of the inferior pedicle, traversing nerve root, and exiting nerve root).[21] Then proceed to open the lateral foramen using the 2-mm cutting burr and 2-mm Kerrison rongeur to remove residual bone, remove the disc and decompress the exiting nerve root and sensory ganglion. The lateral facetectomy is enlarged medial to allow access space for placement of the interbody cage.
- When discectomy is completed, the operating microscope may be removed and surgical loupes used for the remainder of the procedure to accommodate the longer fixation and fusion instruments. The endplates are prepared by scraping and removal. Then interbody spacers are impacted at approximately a

40-degree angle to the midline. The size for interbody cage is determined by the final spacer size accepted. The interbody cage is packed with autograft, either local or harvested from the iliac crest (requires separate incision).

- The interbody cage is impacted and final position is confirmed with biplane fluoroscopy (▶ Fig. 8.6d). Monitoring progress of the cage insertion with intermittent lateral fluoroscopy is useful and a final AP view is essential to confirm optimal medial to lateral position of the implant.
- Then the working tube is expanded to provide pedicle-to-pedicle exposure and the pedicle screw entry point is determined at the junction of the medial transverse process and pars. The transverse process and pars is decorticated with the drill in preparation for the lateral fusion. After completion of interbody cage placement and pedicle screw site exposure, a local anesthetic and steroid-soaked fat graft placed over the sensory ganglion of the exiting nerve root prior to closing will reduce postoperative radicular pain. If more medial unilateral decompression is required, a complete foraminotomy, followed by hemilaminectomy and ligamentum flavectomy will fully expose the exiting and traversing nerve roots and allow removal of canal pathology such as extruded disc or osteophytes with visualization enhanced by the operating microscope.
- After decompression is completed, attention is turned to pedicle screw placement. The entry points are drilled and markers placed, followed by AP and lateral fluoroscopy to confirm proper pedicle placement and initial trajectory. Since tube placement is usually at 30- to 40-degree angle, the pedicle tap and screws can usually be placed directly through the working tube without major trajectory adjustments. Biplane fluoroscopy should be utilized intermittently during the screw placement process to be certain trajectory

and screw depth is correct without need for multiple revisions. The rod is passed directly through the tube, then placed in the screw heads under direct vision. Compression of the screw heads on the rod is essential to prevent backing out laterally of the interbody cage ("close the door when you leave"). Provisional and final tightening of set screws is then performed directly through the working tube. Bone graft can be placed laterally for fusion. After completion of the procedure the tube may be removed, then the fascial layer closed with resorbable suture followed by a subcuticular layer.

- When the ipsilateral side is completed, the contralateral tube placement is performed to expose the transverse processes, pars, and lateral facets to allow decortication and lateral fusion. When performing the TLIF, only one transverse interbody cage is placed from the ipsilateral side. Performing each side separately facilitates fluoroscopic visualization by reducing side-to-side confusion on the lateral views. However, in cases with narrow disc spaces that will not distract adequately with the interbody spacers and bullet nose cages, the contralateral pedicle screws may be placed to allow distraction on the screws to keep the disc space open while placing the ipsilateral cage. Decompression of the contralateral foramen or spinal canal can be performed as on the ipsilateral side. Pedicle screws are then placed in the same manner as on the ipsilateral side remembering to compress the screw heads on the rod before final tightening. Bilateral rather than unilateral pedicle screws are recommended to reduce stress on the pedicle screws and to increase the fusion rate. The contralateral wound is closed as previously described. When the cages and pedicle screws have all been placed, biplane fluoroscopy (or CT) should be performed to confirm all hardware is properly positioned before the patient leaves the operating table.

Complications of Minimally Invasive Surgery Fusion

Some complications of MIS fusion surgery are similar to those encountered during MIS decompression surgery including infection, bleeding, dural tear with CSF leak, and nerve root injury. There are additional issues specific to the fixation techniques that must be considered to prevent complications.

- Bleeding must be meticulously controlled as encountered in order to allow visualization in the working tube. Since bleeding must be controlled to perform the operation, postoperative hematomas are rare. However, use of the expandable tubes to gain exposure increases the risk of bleeding relative to decompression procedures.
- Infection prophylaxis with broad spectrum perioperative antibiotics combined with meticulous sterile technique will reduce the incidence of infection to a minimum. Infection rates should be less than 3% if the perioperative antibiotics cover both gram-positive and gram-negative organisms.
- Dural tears during discectomy or foraminotomy may occur when operating around the thecal sac. The dura must be retracted with a right-angled suction retractor since conventional retractors will block visualization especially when there is significant epidural bleeding. If a dural tear occurs, there is often not enough room in the tube to perform primary suture of the dura, so the repair method consists of application of a synthetic collagen or fascial patch covered by fibrin sealant and reinforced by muscle or fat. A significant or persistent CSF leak will require a lumbar subarachnoid drain for CSF diversion. Failure to adequately stop a CSF leak should not be ignored since the leak increases the risk of infection and meningitis. A persistent leak may require a direct suture repair via open surgery. Dural tear risk is 5 to 10% depending of the surgeon's experience.
- Dural penetration may occur during the dilation process. There is significant risk during the dilation process that requires docking the guidewire under fluoroscopy, then passing small-diameter inner dilators blindly over the guidewire. It is essential to monitor this process with lateral fluoroscopy so the guidewire does not bind to the inner dilator and get pushed through the interlaminar space or into the neuroforamen puncturing or compressing the dura and potentially injuring nerve roots.
- The risk of pseudarthrosis and cage migration has been determined to be unacceptably high with stand-alone interbody cages. Therefore, the use of pedicle fixation (TLIF, PLIF) or direct plating of the interspace (XLIF) is required to prevent this complication. In selected cases without instability, unilateral fixation may be satisfactory.
- Prevention of cage migration also requires compression of pedicle screws to "close the door" and prevent the cages from moving out of the interspace into the canal or foramen where they may cause nerve root compression. If such migration occurs, replacement or removal of the cage is necessary as soon possible to prevent scarring to the nerve root and bone fusion healing that would make the later revision more difficult and likely to cause an irreversible nerve root injury and chronic pain. Misplaced pedicle screws breaching the medial pedicle and impinging on nerve roots in the adjacent foramen or thecal sac must be recognized and removed as soon as possible. A CT scan should be performed prior to discharge to confirm good cage and pedicle screw placement. Delay to remove the offending pedicle screws may lead to development of an irreversible chronic complex regional pain syndrome even in the absence of overt radiculopathy.

- The use of bone morphogenetic protein (BMP) to enhance osteogenesis within disc space and interbody cages placed via the posterolateral approach carries with it the risk of ectopic bone formation encasing the adjacent nerve roots Therefore, if BMP is used, it should be delivered via a tube placed in the anterior disc space and completely emptied with a stylet prior to removal to prevent BMP leakage into the epidural space. Placing a BMP-soaked pledget within the cage will insure leakage into the epidural space when impacting the cage into the interspace. Ectopic bone formation around nerve roots will cause an irreversible chronic radicular pain syndrome.

8.5.2 Posterior Lumbar Interbody Fusion

Introduction

The PLIF approach is similar to the TLIF except that it is centered at the medial foramen rather than the lateral foramen and includes a lateral laminectomy for interbody placement (▶ Fig. 8.7a). The MIS approach to spinal fusion requires a larger exposure than the decompression surgery. The tubes placed for pedicle screw fixation (currently the standard of care for spinal fusion due to high fixation rates) must expand in the muscle to allow pedicle to pedicle exposure. Some have claimed that the need for expandable tubes means the approach is no longer MIS, but "mini-open." However, even considering the tube expansion the MIS PLIF as described is less invasive than methods requiring four to six incisions of 2 cm length to allow "percutaneous" pedicle screw placement.[22,29] There is little difference in exposure when bilateral tubular exposure is compared with unilateral tube and contralateral percutaneous pedicle screw fixation except that contralateral fusion is not possible with the latter weakening the fusion construct. The more medial PLIF approach allows more direct access to the spinal canal pathology, but carries with it the risk of over-retraction of the thecal sac and cauda equina injury when placing interbody cages. Since the canal is wider at the L5–S1 level than the other lumbar disc levels, over-retraction is less likely than at higher levels where the TLIF approach is safer (▶ Fig. 8.7b).

Clinical Presentation

- Painful radiculopathy of L5 or S1 with low back pain.
- Incapacitating antigravity axial chronic low back pain due to L5–S1 degenerative discs.

Image Pathology

- Evidence of excessive vertebral motion ("instability") contributory to symptomatology.
- Severe degenerative discogenic changes contributory to axial antigravity pain (L5–S1).

Contraindications (Relative)

- The MIS PLIF approach is applicable mainly for single-level pathology at L5–S1.
- Fusions of more than one level.
- High-grade spondylolisthesis.
- Central canal stenosis bilateral and greater than 2 cm length.

Operative Technique

The operative technique (▶ Fig. 8.7)[22,29] is bilateral flank incisions (2–2.5 cm laterally) at L5–S1 (3.0–3.6 cm length) tube size (28–34 mm).

- After induction of general endotracheal anesthesia, the patient is placed prone on a spinal frame and the back prepped and draped in the standard manner. The bilateral incision size should be 2 mm greater than the anticipated working tube diameter.

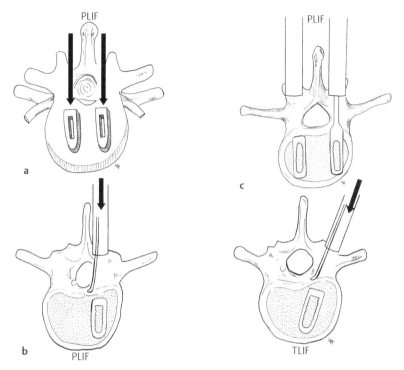

Fig. 8.7 **(a)** Trajectory for placement of PLIF interbody cage. **(b)** Comparison of thecal sac retraction necessary for PLIF compared to TLIF **(c)** MIS tube placements for bilateral PLIF.

- Place a 22-gauge spinal needle in the center of the anticipated incision sites to the depth of the medial facet. Note the level of needle insertion to assure it correlates with the imaging and pathological condition. Use biplane fluoroscopy to accurately determine the required tube length and trajectory. Measure the final depth of the needle to confirm the tube length.
- Make the skin incision (3–3.6 cm) only after absolute certainty that the proper level, trajectory, and position with respect to the surgical pathology have been determined about 2 cm lateral (▶ Fig. 8.7a). Dissect to the level of the fascia and open to the same width as the skin incision 5 to 10 mm greater than the working tube diameter to accommodate expansion.
- Place the guidewire to the level of the medial facet and dock in bone, making

certain that the docking site is not too near the interlaminar space to avoid the penetrating the dura and nerve root, and confirm its position with biplane fluoroscopy. Pass the inner dilator over the guidewire rotating the dilator until it hits the medial facet. Then again confirm that the guidewire and dilator are properly positioned using biplane fluoroscopy before proceeding with dilation. Pass additional dilators until the desired working diameter is achieved 28 to 34 mm depending on the pathology. The working tube should be expandable (50–60 mm) to allow pedicle-to-pedicle exposure. The operating microscope will then be positioned to allow illumination and visualization of the operative site at the bottom of the tube.
- At this point, after removing residual subcutaneous tissue, a 2-mm cutting

115

burr is used to thin the laminectomy and medial facet. The residual bone is then removed with a 2-mm Kerrison rongeur. The ligamentum flavum is then removed and the disc space and S1 nerve root identified. An L5–S1 discectomy is performed protecting the S1 nerve root with a suction retractor. The laminotomy and L5 foraminotomy are enlarged laterally to allow access space for placement of the interbody cage. When the discectomy and lateral exposure is completed, the operating microscope is removed. Under loupe magnification, the endplates are prepared by scraping and removal. Bone graft material is placed through a funnel into the anterior disc space for fusion after the disc space is empty.

- Extreme care must be taken not to allow over-retraction of the thecal sac medially (< 50%) by leaving some midline lamina to block the retractor pull medially (▶ Fig. 8.7b). Then sequential size interbody spacers are impacted at approximately a 20-degree angle to the midline. The size for the interbody cage is determined by the final spacer size accepted. However, in cases with narrow disc spaces that will not distract adequately with the interbody spacers and bullet nose cages, the contralateral pedicle screws may be placed to allow distraction on the screws to keep the disc space open while placing the ipsilateral cage.

- The interbody cage is packed with autograft either local or harvested from the iliac crest (may be harvested prior to tube placement from the same incision). The interbody cage is impacted and final position is confirmed with biplane fluoroscopy (or CT). Monitoring progress of the cage insertion with intermittent lateral fluoroscopy is useful and a final AP view is essential to confirm optimal medial to lateral position of the implant.

- When the ipsilateral side is completed, the contralateral tube placement is performed to expose the lamina and facet

for discectomy and fusion. When a PLIF discectomy is performed, bilateral interbody cages are placed vertically on each side, not transversely as for the TLIF (▶ Fig. 8.7c). Performing each side separately facilitates fluoroscopic visualization by reducing side-to-side confusion on the lateral views. Pedicle screws are then placed in the same manner as on the ipsilateral side remembering to compress the screw heads on the rod before final tightening. Bilateral rather than unilateral interbody cages and pedicle screws are recommended to reduce stress on the pedicle screws and to increase the fusion rate. The contralateral wound is closed as previously described. When the cages and pedicle screws have been placed, biplane fluoroscopy (or CT) should be performed to confirm all hardware is properly positioned before the patient leaves the operating table.

Complications

- Bleeding and epidural hematoma.
- Infection and discitis.
- Dural tear with CSF leak.
- Pseudarthrosis.
- Cage migration out of the disc space.
- Misplaced pedicle screws.
- Ectopic bone with BMP.
- Cauda equina injury due to over-retraction.

8.5.3 Extreme Lumbar Interbody Fusion

Introduction

The XLIF approach is different from the TLIF and PLIF since it is centered at the midpoint of the lateral vertebral body with the incision in the flank and a long tubular retractor passed unilaterally through the psoas muscle adjacent to the vertebrae (▶ Fig. 8.8a, b). The MIS approach to spinal fusion requires a larger exposure than the decompression surgery and with the longer distance traversed by the XLIF tube, this approach is more invasive than the TLIF or XLIF. In addition, the XLIF lateral approach introduces safety issues associated with the technique. Passage of the working tube laterally through the psoas muscle carries with it the risk of psoas muscle injury and nerve damage to branches of the lumbar plexus within the psoas resulting in new pain and weakness in the ipsilateral lower extremity.[30] In order to mitigate this risk, neuromonitoring is required to detect retractor-related nerve injury whenever the XLIF approach is utilized. In addition, lateral vertebral plates or percutaneous pedicle or facet screws are recommended to add stability to the fused segments and this requires additional lateral or posterior exposure. The XLIF fusion may be used L1–L2 to L4–L5 for interbody multilevel fusions with two levels approached through a single skin incision, but separate subcutaneous trajectories. The XLIF is capable of indirectly decompressing nerve roots compressed in the foramen by increasing the foramen size with insertion of the interbody cage, but will not directly treat pathology within the spinal canal.[31] This latter fact, the inability to directly decompress nerve roots, greatly restricts the utility of the XLIF approach for treatment of patients with radiculopathy. The advantage of the XLIF is that multiple levels of the lumbar spine can be treated for anterior correction of deformity as well as indirect enlargement of foramina. Monitoring the procedure with fluoroscopy is essential, but due to the table position, intraoperative CT scanning is not used (if available) until the procedure is completed.

Clinical Presentation

- Painful radiculopathy of L1–L5.
- Incapacitating antigravity axial chronic low back pain due to L1–L5 degenerative discs.
- Lumbar degenerative scoliosis or kyphosis.
- Lumbar spondylolisthesis grade 1.

Image Pathology

- Evidence of excessive vertebral motion ("instability") contributory to symptomatology.
- Severe degenerative discogenic changes contributory to axial antigravity pain (L1–L5).

Contraindications (Relative)

- The MIS XLIF approach is not applicable at L5–S1 due to approach block by the ileum.
- High-grade spondylolisthesis requiring direct reduction.
- Central canal stenosis or disc herniation not relieved by indirect decompression.

Operative Technique

The operative technique (▶ Fig. 8.8)[32,33,34,35] is unilateral flank incision (20–30 cm laterally) at L1–L5 (4–5 cm length) tube size (30–45 mm).

- After induction of general endotracheal anesthesia the patient is placed in the lateral decubitus position on a radiolucent operating table with the table flexed to increase the distance between the rib cage margin and the iliac crest. The back and entire flank is prepped and draped in the standard manner. The fluoroscope is positioned so that AP and lateral images can be obtained intraoperatively. The flank incision should be directly lateral to the fusion level as seen on the lateral view, and the incision size should be 2 mm greater than the anticipated working tube diameter (▶ Fig. 8.8a). The distance to midline posteriorly is not used due to the variation of waist size. A second posterolateral incision is used by some surgeons to guide the working tube in the retroperitoneal space with finger dissection in order to avoid bowel or kidney injury.
- Place the inner dilator in the center of the incision site to the depth of the psoas muscle. Note the trajectory of the dilator

117

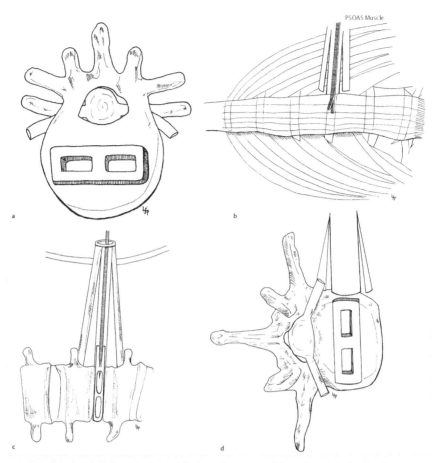

Fig. 8.8 (a) Trajectory for placement of XLIF interbody cage. **(b)** MIS lateral flank tube placement and XLIF discectomy. **(c)** Trial spacer insertion for determination of cage size. **(d)** Final position of the XLIF interbody device and working tube.

on insertion with biplane fluoroscopy to assure it correlates with the imaging and pathological levels. Measure the insertion length to determine the required working tube length.

- The XLIF dilators have embedded stimulating electrodes for EMG (electromyographic) monitoring in the lower extremities to decrease retractor injury to lumbar plexus nerves during passage through the psoas muscle. Entry into the psoas muscle should be at the junction of the anterior and middle third of the muscle to minimize the risk of nerve injury.

- Pass the inner dilator to the midportion of the lateral disc space and confirm the location with biplane fluoroscopy. Pass additional dilators until the desired working diameter is achieved 28 to 34 mm depending on the pathology. The radiolucent expandable working tube should then be passed flush with the lateral vertebral bodies and centered on the disc space (▶ Fig. 8.8b).

- The operating microscope will then be positioned to allow illumination and visualization of the operative site at the bottom of the tube. At this point, after removing residual subcutaneous tissue, a lateral annulotomy is performed and the complete discectomy is performed with pituitary rongeurs and angled curettes (▶ Fig. 8.8b). When the discectomy and lateral exposure is completed, the operating microscope is removed. Under loupe magnification, the endplates should be decorticated, but not destroyed, to prevent interbody subsidence into the vertebral body. The contralateral annulus is released with a Cobb elevator passed through the disc space to allow access for distraction and placement of the interbody cage. Then the appropriate size cage is determined with trial spacers. The cage is selected for insertion. Under biplane fluoroscopy, the implant is positioned at the junction of the anterior and middle third of the disc space on the lateral view and passed from the outer portion of the vertebral rim on each side under AP fluoroscopy (▶ Fig. 8.8c, d).
- Supplemental lateral plate and screws may be used for additional fixation using the expandable tube to allow increased cephalad–caudal exposure. Posterior fixation with percutaneous pedicle or facet screws is an alternative option to the lateral plate, but requires other incisions for the posterior approach effectively disqualifying the procedure as MIS.
- After completion of the interbody cage insertion and plate fixation, the working tube may be removed, then the fascial layer, and then closed with resorbable suture, followed by a subcutaneous and subcuticular layer.

Complications

- Bleeding with psoas and retroperitoneal hematoma.
- Infection.
- Ipsilateral hip flexion (psoas) weakness and pain.
- Injury to the vena cava or aorta anterior to the spine.
- Kidney or ureter/bowel injury.
- Nerve root injury and posterior encroachment on the spinal canal.
- Lumbar plexus injury causing weakness and pain.
- Cage subsidence, breakage, misplacement, migration.
- Pseudarthrosis or vertebral body fracture.

8.6 Advantages and Disadvantages of MIS versus Open Techniques

8.6.1 Advantages

- A smaller exposure equates with less pain resulting in faster mobilization, lower narcotic requirement, and shorter length of stay in the hospital such that the procedures can be confidently and safely performed on an outpatient basis.
- A smaller exposure heals more rapidly with fewer wound problems especially in the obese patient with deep subcutaneous tissue. The smaller incisions also have a lower infection rate related to the decreased exposed operative area.
- Blood loss is reduced markedly compared with open procedures.
- Outcomes and complications are similar to those of traditional open procedures.[36]
- Shorter length of stay and more rapid mobilization with comparable outcomes equates to lower costs, earlier return to work, and increased value of the surgery to patients.
- Minimizing the exposure to that which allows safely accomplishing the surgical goal is as "simple as possible" and is the essence of MIS.

8.6.2 Disadvantages

- An MIS approach is technically challenging especially for surgeons trained only with the open technique. The learning curve is steeper than for the open surgery and the potential for errors related to improper tube placement and guidewires entering the spinal canal increases risks. Concern over technical matters often increases the duration of MIS procedures compared to their open counterparts. It is essential that surgeons be trained in the open spine procedures prior to attempting the minimally invasive approach.
- Dural tears are the most common complications with MIS surgery and these are difficult to repair due to the technical difficulty of suture repair and may require CSF diversion or reoperation via an open approach.
- The potential to perform an inadequate surgery related to limited exposure of pathology is a significant risk of the MIS approach.
- Consider the advantages and disadvantages of the competing approaches, which differ depending on the patient and the pathology, in order to achieve the best outcome.
- Reducing exposure to less than that required for an optimal outcome is "simpler than possible." Knowing the right exposure for the pathology is the art of lumbar spine MIS.

8.6.3 The Future of Minimally Invasive Surgery for the Lumbar Spine

- The number of spine MIS procedures is rapidly increasing with the expectation that by 2020 more than half of all spine surgeries will be performed with minimally invasive techniques.[37]
- Technology is always improving such that what seems impossible today will be possible tomorrow. The role of MIS in more complex spine pathology such as adult degenerative deformity is yet to be determined.[38,39,40]
- MIS surgery is proving to have decreased cost than the traditional open surgery with equivalent clinical outcomes.[26,27,36] Due to the aging population and increasing incidence of lumbar spine degeneration in the population, high-value treatments are being sought to reduce the societal cost burden. This issue will be a major factor resulting in increased utilization of MIS spine surgery in the future.

References

[1] Foley KT, Smith MM. Microendoscopic discectomy. Tech Neurosurg. 1997; 3:301–307

[2] Wiltse LL. The paraspinal sacrospinalis-splitting approach to the lumbar spine. Clin Orthop Relat Res. 1973(91):48–57

[3] Kim CW. Scientific basis of minimally invasive spine surgery: prevention of multifidus muscle injury during posterior lumbar surgery. Spine. 2010; 35(26) Suppl:S281–S286

[4] McAfee PC, Phillips FM, Andersson G, et al. Minimally invasive spine surgery. Spine. 2010; 35(26) Suppl:S271–S273

[5] Dasenbrock HH, Juraschek SP, Schultz LR, et al. The efficacy of minimally invasive discectomy compared with open discectomy: a meta-analysis of prospective randomized controlled trials. J Neurosurg Spine. 2012; 16(5):452–462

[6] Perez-Cruet MJ, Foley KT, Isaacs RE, et al. Microendendoscopic lumbar discectomy: technical note. Neurosurgery. 2002; 51(5):146–154

[7] Perez-Cruet MJ, Fessler RG, Perin NI. Review: complications of minimally invasive spinal surgery. Neurosurgery. 2002; 51(5) Suppl:S26–S36

[8] O'Toole JE, Eichholz KM, Fessler RG. Surgical site infection rates after minimally invasive spinal surgery. J Neurosurg Spine. 2009; 11(4):471–476

[9] Khoo LT, Fessler RG. Microendoscopic decompression laminotomy for treatment of lumbar stenosis. Neurosurgery. 2002; 51(5):129–136

[10] Guiot BH, Khoo LT, Fessler RG. A minimally invasive technique for decompression of the lumbar spine. Spine. 2002; 27(4):432–438

[11] Popov V, Anderson DG. Minimal invasive decompression for lumbar spinal stenosis. Adv Orthop. 2012; 2012:6453211

[12] Palmer S, Turner R, Palmer R. Bilateral decompression of lumbar spinal stenosis involving a unilateral approach with microscope and tubular retractor system. J Neurosurg. 2002; 97(2) Suppl:213–217

[13] Boukebir M, Berlin CD, Hartl R, et al. Ten-Step MIS Lumbar Decompression and Dural Repair through Tubular Retractors. Operative Neurosurgery. 2017; 13(2):232–245

[14] Alimi M, Hofstetter CP, Pyo SY, Paulo D, Härtl R. Minimally invasive laminectomy for lumbar spinal stenosis in patients with and without preoperative spondylolisthesis: clinical outcome and reoperation rates. J Neurosurg Spine. 2015; 22(4):339–352

[15] Phan K, Dunn AE, Rao PJ, Mobbs RJ. Far lateral microdiscectomy: a minimally-invasive surgical technique for the treatment of far lateral lumbar disc herniation. J Spine Surg. 2016; 2(1):59–63

[16] Kotil K, Akcetin M, Bilge T. A minimally invasive transmuscular approach to far-lateral L5-S1 level disc herniations: a prospective study. J Spinal Disord Tech. 2007; 20(2):132–138

[17] Foley KT, Smith MM, Rampersaud YR. Microendoscopic approach to far-lateral lumbar disc herniation. Neurosurg Focus. 1999; 7(5):e5

[18] Kambin P, Zhou L. History and current status of percutaneous arthroscopic disc surgery. Spine. 1996; 21(24) Suppl:57S–61S

[19] Meyer SA, Wu J-C, Mummaneni PV. Mini-open and minimally invasive transforaminal lumbar interbody fusion: technique review. Semin Spine Surg. 2011; 23:45–50

[20] Foley KT, Holly LT, Schwender JD. Minimally invasive lumbar fusion. Spine. 2003; 28(15) Suppl: S26–S35

[21] Hardenbrook M, Lombardo S, Wilson MC, Telfeian AE. The anatomic rationale for transforaminal endoscopic interbody fusion: a cadaveric analysis. Neurosurg Focus. 2016; 40(2):E12

[22] German JW, Foley KT. Minimal access surgical techniques in the management of the painful lumbar motion segment. Spine. 2005; 30(16) Suppl: S52–S59

[23] Sandhu FA, Voyadzis J-M, Fessler RG. Lumbar Spine. Decision Making for Minimally Invasive Spine Surgery. New York, NY:Thieme; 2011; Section III: Chapters 7-10:91-146

[24] Wu RH, Fraser JF, Härtl R. Minimal access versus open transforaminal lumbar interbody fusion: meta-analysis of fusion rates. Spine. 2010; 35 (26):2273–2281

[25] Dhall SS, Wang MY, Mummaneni PV. Clinical and radiographic comparison of mini-open transforaminal interbody fusion with open TLIF in 42 patients with long-term follow-up. J Neurosurg Spine. 2008; 9(6):560–565

[26] Goldstein CL, Phillips FM, Rampersaud YR. Comparative effectiveness and economic evaluations of open versus minimally invasive posterior or transforaminal lumbar interbody fusion: a systematic review. Spine. 2016; 41 Suppl 8:S74–S89

[27] McGirt MJ, Parker SL, Mummaneni P, et al. Is the use of minimally invasive fusion technologies associated with improved outcomes after elective interbody lumbar fusion? Analysis of a nationwide prospective patient-reported outcomes registry. Spine J. 2017; 17(7):922–932

[28] Karikari IO, Isaacs RE. Minimally invasive transforaminal lumbar interbody fusion: a review of techniques and outcomes. Spine. 2010; 35(26) Suppl: S294–S301

[29] Khoo LT, Palmer S, Laich DT, Fessler RG. Minimally invasive percutaneous posterior lumbar interbody fusion. Neurosurgery. 2002; 51(5) Suppl:S166–S181

[30] Smith WD, Wohns RNW, Christian G, Rodgers EJ, Rodgers WB. Outpatient minimally invasive lumbar interbody fusion predictive factors and clinical results. Spine. 2016; 41 Suppl 8:S106–S122

[31] Oliveira L, Marchi L, Coutinho E, Pimenta L. A radiographic assessment of the ability of the extreme lateral interbody fusion procedure to indirectly decompress the neural elements. Spine. 2010; 35(26) Suppl:S331–S337

[32] Ozgur BM, Aryan HE, Pimenta L, Taylor WR. Extreme Lateral Interbody Fusion (XLIF): a novel surgical technique for anterior lumbar interbody fusion. Spine J. 2006; 6(4):435–443

[33] Billinghurst J, Akbarnis BA. Extreme lateral interbody fusion – XLIF. Curr Orthop Pract. 2009; 20 (3):238–251

[34] Youssef JA, McAfee PC, Patty CA, et al. Minimally invasive surgery: lateral approach interbody fusion: results and review. Spine. 2010; 35(26) Suppl:S302–S311

[35] Yen CP, Uribe JS. Procedural checklist for retroperitoneal transpsoas minimally invasive lateral interbody fusion. Spine. 2016; 41 Suppl 8:S152–S158

[36] Lu VM, Kerezoudis P, Gilder HE, McCutcheon BA, Phan K, Bydon M. Minimally invasive surgery versus open surgery spinal fusion for spondylolisthesis. Spine. 2017; 42(3):E177–E185

[37] Phillips FM, Cheng I, Rampersaud YR, et al. Breaking through the "glass ceiling" of minimally invasive spine surgery. Spine. 2016; 41 Suppl 8:S39–S43

[38] Savage JW. The optimal treatment for symptomatic neurogenic claudication or radiculopathy in the presence of mild degenerative scoliosis remains unclear. Spine J. 2017; 17(1):44–45

[39] Goldstein CL, Macwan K, Sundararajan K, Rampersaud YR. Perioperative outcomes and adverse events of minimally invasive versus open posterior lumbar fusion: meta-analysis and systematic review. J Neurosurg Spine. 2016; 24(3):416–427

[40] Tay KS, Bassi A, Yeo W, Yue WM. Associated lumbar scoliosis does not affect outcomes in patients undergoing focal minimally invasive surgery-transforaminal lumbar interbody fusion (MISTLIF) for neurogenic symptoms-a minimum 2-year follow-up study. Spine J. 2017; 17(1):34–43

9 Postoperative Care

Abstract

The control of postoperative pain in the initial 48 hours is especially critical in patients having undergone more extensive surgery requiring instrumentation. Otherwise, the patient may experience a psychological stress that can result in a very deleterious effect on eventual outcome.

The multi-modal approach to pain control will decrease narcotic usage. Pre-emptive medication(e.g. gabapentin) within this regimen should be considered. Nonsteroidal anti-inflammatory drugs (NSAIDs) are very effective postoperatively as well. But they can effect bone healing and selective Cox 2 inhibitors (e.g. diclofenac, meloxicam] should be avoided. Non-selective Cox inhibitors (e.g. ketorolac, ibuprofen, naproxen] may be used in first 48 hours postoperatively. Acetaminophen (paracetamol) has weak Cox inhibition and has become the drug of choice.

An open surgical wound presents as an opportunity for placement of catheter for postoperative epidural analgesia (PEA). This technique can result in dramatic results, but its general advantage over patient-controlled IV analgesia (PCIA) has not been conclusively shown; technical issues are likely factors in this measured equivalency. One main drawback with PEA is the potential for root desensitization when an anesthetic is used, with a confounding postoperative motor weakness.

Postoperative infection control is afforded by a meticulous closure technique. As many, if not most, infections begin superficially (subcutaneously) then attention to well-apposed skin edges is mandatory. Drains should be used liberally and should always exit at the cranial end of the incision, away from anal contamination.

The duration of postoperative antibiotics should be individualized. The rate of postoperative infection has been consistently shown to be related to the duration of surgery; hence, the duration of postoperative antibiotics dosage should reflect this time-related contamination potential.

Keywords: multi-modal pain control, Cox inhibition, postoperative epidural analgesia (PEA), antibiotic powder, lymphocyte count, C-reactive protein

9.1 Systemic Pain Control

9.1.1 Introduction

In most cases of decompressive degenerative spine surgery, routine intravenous (IV) and oral regimens are adequate for postoperative pain control. More extensive surgeries, especially those requiring instrumentation, require a concerted effort to avoid significant postoperative pain, especially in the first 48 hours. It is critical in this period that the patient avoids a pain traumatization that can later cause psychological consequences with considerable effect on patient outcome. But it also must be emphasized that analgesia is a significant cause of perioperative mortality, especially in young and middle-aged patients.[1]

9.1.2 Multimodal Approach[2,3,4,5]

Preemptive Non-narcotics: The reduction of narcotic usage postoperatively can be considered a measure of better pain control and improved quality of life. Non-narcotic regimens with *preemptive* dosage have been shown to be effective in this regard. These medications include the following:

- Gabapentin/pregabalin (oral).[6,7]
- Nonsteroidal anti-inflammatory drugs (NSAIDs).[8,9]

○ Nonselective cyclooxygenase (Cox) inhibitors: ibuprofen, ketorolac, indomethacin, piroxicam, naproxen.

○ Selective Cox-2 inhibitors: "Coxibs," endolac, meloxicam, diclofenac.

○ Weak Cox inhibition: acetaminophen (paracetamol).

NSAIDs and Analgesia: Studies have shown that NSAIDs are at least as effective as opiates for pain control after bony fracture or postoperatively after fixation. These drugs, furthermore, avoid the negative side effects of opiates: respiratory depression, sedation, cognitive slowing. The use of IV acetaminophen and ibuprofen peri- and postoperatively has been shown to be effective and relatively safe in nonspinal cases.[10] The reluctance in their use in the setting of bone fracture is related to evidence that they have a negative effect on bone healing.[11]

9.1.3 Effect of NSAIDs on Bone Healing/Fusion [8,9,12]

These medications affect the antipyretic, analgesic, and anti-inflammatory properties by inhibition of enzymatic (Cox) production of prostaglandins.[13] After a fracture, there is evidence that the Cox-2 enzymatic prostaglandin release plays a critical role in the induction of osteoblasts in the early stage of bone healing. The effect of prostaglandins on bone cells is unclear, but it may be related to the expression of the bone morphogenic protein (BMP). Selective Cox-1 inhibition does not seem to have a similar effect.

Clinical studies on the effect of NSAIDs on bone healing and spinal fusion are conflicting. Some studies suggest no effect on postfusion union rates,[14,15] while others show a dose-dependent inhibitory effect.[16,17,18] These studies analyze various NSAIDs, dose regimens, duration of usage, and subject age variances; thus, no definitive general conclusions can be drawn from these uncontrolled studies. However, with the established biochemistry, and with and the results of in vitro and animal model studies, caution is warranted in the use of Cox inhibitory NSAIDs after spinal fusion.

Acetaminophen: As acetaminophen is a weak Cox inhibitor, it has minimal effect on prostaglandin synthesis. There are no studies demonstrating a significantly negative effect on bone healing and/or fusion. In one animal study, the acute treatment of acetaminophen had no effect on fracture healing, contrasting with a significantly higher nonunion rate in celecoxib-treated animals.[19]

Acetaminophen is thus the logical choice for NSAID use in perioperative setting.[20] The availability of an IV form removes problematic issues of oral intake in this period.

9.1.4 Conclusion

• Perioperative nonnarcotic medications reduce opiate use for postoperative pain control, thus diminishing the negative side effects of narcotics, and with greater patient satisfaction.

• Gabapentin (1,200 mg/d) or pregabalin (300 mg/d) has opiate sparing effect if administered from 12 hours preoperatively to 12 to 24 hours postoperatively.

• NSAIDs similarly can be effectively added to a *multimodal* regimen.

• Because Cox inhibition (with subsequent diminished prostaglandin production) has been shown to be associated with decreased bone healing and fusion, *selective* Cox-2 inhibitory NSAIDs should be avoided for perioperative pain control in cases involving bony arthrodesis. In the acute postoperative period (24–48 hours), *nonselective* Cox inhibitors may be an effective alternative to acetaminophen.

• Acetaminophen is the NSAID of choice for adjutant acute pain control when bony fusion is desired (1 g IV intraoperatively and 1 g IV every 6–8 hours for 24–48 hours postoperatively).

9.2 Postoperative Epidural Analgesia

The use of epidural analgesia after nonspinal abdominal and thoracic surgeries has been proven to be of significant benefit.[21, 22] Similar benefits after spinal surgery would seem a logical extrapolation, especially as the open surgical field allows for direct placement of the epidural catheter. The value of postoperative epidural analgesia (PEA) may be proportional to the anticipated stress response of the surgery.[23]

Single bolus epidural fentanyl has been shown to be effective.[24,25] The use of PEA via indwelling catheter remains *controversial*. Controlled studies report conflicting conclusions as to the efficacy of pain control in patients with patient-controlled epidural analgesia (PCEA) versus patient-controlled IV analgesia (PCIA).[26,27,28] Furthermore, the potential for epidural medication to confound the postoperative neurological exam (with the possibility of masking neurologic compromise from an epidural hematoma) has prevented a wider acceptance of this technique.[29]

The published efficacy of PEA is difficult to interpret due to the variability in the regimens/dosages, techniques, and outcome measurement.

9.2.1 Regimens/Dosages

- Intraoperative bolus optional.
- Infusion control: continuous infusion, patient controlled, both.
- Duration of infusion: 1 to 4 days.
- Onset of infusion: immediately in postanesthesia care unit (PACU) or after patient awakes following a neurologic examination.
- Infusion regimen: narcotic, anesthetic, both; variable rates of infusion.
- Narcotic infusion: fentanyl, sufentanil, morphine.

- Anesthetic infusion: bupivacaine, ropivacaine

9.2.2 Techniques

- Placement of catheter: at site of surgery, varying distance cephalad of site.
- Catheter: diameter, rigidity, aperture configuration.
- With or without radiographic confirmation of catheter position.

9.2.3 Outcomes Assessment

- Patient assessment: VAS (visual analog scale), subjective.
- Functional capabilities: turning in bed, time to ambulation, length of hospital stay.
- Supplementary narcotic usage.
- Side effects: hypotension, respiratory depression, anesthetic neurologic deficit.

9.2.4 Conclusion

In conclusion, the absence of conformity in published study design allows limited conclusion as to the evidence of significant advantage of PEA over PCIA. Furthermore, major complications are reported.[30] However, there have been relatively consistent findings:

The efficacy of pain control of PEA has not been shown to be inferior to PCIA and in some studies has been shown to be superior.[31]

PEA patients require less systemic narcotics (with subsequent potential advantages in regard to sedation and mobilization).

The temporary side effects pose increased postoperative care issues needing attention by surgeon and nursing staff, mainly hypotension and motor/sensory deficit.

Neurologic side effects (primarily motor weakness) have posed a major drawback for surgical use of PEA.

There have been no studies comparing the long-term outcomes of PCIA versus PEA.

9.3 Infection Control

9.3.1 Introduction

The postoperative morbidity of surgical site infections is well established.[32] There is evidence that the patient's skin is a source of intraoperative inoculation, and a significant number of postoperative deep space infections begin superficially (subcutaneously).[33]

9.3.2 Risk Factors[34,35,36]

- Duration of surgery of greater than 3 hours.
- Insulin-dependent diabetes mellitus: preoperative A1c > 7%.
- ASA (American Society of Anesthesiologists) class of 3.
- Current smoking (risk reduced by cessation).
- Preoperative anemia: hematocrit (HCT) < 36.
- Prior operation.[37]
- Obesity: BMI (body mass index) > 30.
- Nasal methicillin-resistant *Staphylococcus aureus* (MRSA) carriers.

9.3.3 Operative Technique/ Care to Minimize Infection Rate

- Coverage of open implant sets with a sterile towel.[38]
- Frequent irrigation with antibiotic saline solution (bacitracin or gentamycin) during procedure and after each level of closure.
- Methodical ongoing intraoperative hemostasis: postoperative drainage, if necessary, exiting from the cranial end of the wound.
- Changing outer gloves every 2 to 3 hours.
- Meticulous skin closure with well-apposed edges.
- Antibiotic ointment on suture/staple line.

- Dressing change when saturation level prevents further wicking.
- Generous use of blood replacement (and postoperatively) to keep HCT > 30 (authors' preference).

9.3.4 Intrawound Antibiotic Powder

- There is evidence that vancomycin powder locally applied into wound can significantly reduce postoperative infections in instrumented cases[36,39,40,41,42] (though one systemic review suggested otherwise).[43]
- The addition of 0.3% betadine as irrigation solution to vancomycin powder (and with bacteriology assessment) has been shown to be very effective against MRSA.[37]
- One report failed to substantiate the benefit of vancomycin powder.[44]

9.3.5 Antibiotic Prophylaxis

- Pre-incision and every 3 to 4 hours during procedure.
- Duration of postoperative antibiotics is dependent on the duration of surgical wound exposure: recommend giving 12 hours of antibiotics for each hour the surgical wound is open (e.g., for a 6-hour case, antibiotic therapy for 3 days).

9.3.6 Postoperative Systemic Markers

A surgical site infection can be predicted with high degree of sensitivity within 1 week of surgery.[45]

- Lymphocyte count at 4 days postoperatively: < 1,180/μL (90.9% sensitivity, 65.4% specificity).
- Lymphocyte count at 7 days postoperatively: < 1,090/μL (63.6% sensitivity, 78.5% specificity).
- C-reactive protein level at 7 days postoperatively: > 4.4 mg/dL (90.9% sensitivity, 89.2% specificity).

9.3.7 Care of Postoperative Deep Space Infection in Noninstrumented Cases

- Incision, debridement, lavage, and long-term drainage (vacuum assisted).
- Long-term culture (7 days).
- Microbial-guided therapy with IV antibiotic for 6 weeks (or as per infectious disease recommendation).

9.3.8 Care of Postoperative Deep Space Infection in Instrumented Cases

- PET (positron emission tomography)/CT (computed tomography) shown to be effective in identifying surgical site infection in suspected cases despite presence of instrumentation.[46]
- Titanium instrumentation: less predilection than stainless steel for microbial biofilm production; aggressive surgical debridement and microbial-guided pharmacotherapy (with vacuum assisted closure) shown to be 100% successful.[47]
- Implant removal has been advocated with fastidious organisms (e.g., *Propionibacterium*)[48] and delayed development of infection (> 3 month).[49]
- Hyperbaric oxygen is a newer therapeutic approach with promising early results.[50]

9.4 Unknowns and Investigational Opportunities

- Further refinement of postoperative epidural technique: role of patient dosing (PCEA), addition/deletion of anesthetic, narcotic dosages relative to patient drug history.
- Development of epidural catheter design and introduction mechanism.
- Role of postoperative biochemical markers (lymphocyte count and CRP [C-reactive protein]) as directive of prophylactic antibiotic dose extension.

References

[1] Juratli SM, Mirza SK, Fulton-Kehoe D, Wickizer TM, Franklin GM. Mortality after lumbar fusion surgery. Spine. 2009; 34(7):740–747

[2] Devin CJ, McGirt MJ. Best evidence in multimodal pain management in spine surgery and means of assessing postoperative pain and functional outcomes. J Clin Neurosci. 2015; 22(6):930–938

[3] Lee BH, Park JO, Sukis LS, et al. Pre-emptive and multi-modal perioperative pain management may improve quality of life in patients undergoing spinal surgery. Pain Physician. 2013; 16(3):E217–226

[4] Mathiesen O, Dahl B, Thomsen BA, et al. A comprehensive multimodal pain treatment reduces opioid consumption after multilevel spine surgery. Eur Spine J. 2013; 22(9):2089–2096

[5] von der Hoeh NH, Voelker A, Gulow J, Uhle U, Przkora R, Heyde CE. Impact of a multidisciplinary pain program for the management of chronic low back pain in patients undergoing spine surgery and primary total hip replacement: a retrospective cohort study. Patient Saf Surg. 2014; 8(1):34

[6] Khurana G, Jindal P, Sharma JP, Bansal KK. Postoperative pain and long-term functional outcome after administration of gabapentin and pregabalin in patients undergoing spinal surgery. Spine. 2014; 39(6):E363–E368

[7] Radhakrishnan M, Bithal PK, Chaturvedi A. Effect of preemptive gabapentin on postoperative pain relief and morphine consumption following lumbar laminectomy and discectomy: a randomized, double-blinded, placebo-controlled study. J Neurosurg Anesthesiol. 2005; 17(3):125–128

[8] Pountos I, Georgouli T, Calori GM, Giannoudis PV. Do nonsteroidal anti-inflammatory drugs affect bone healing? A critical analysis. Sci World J. 2012; 2012:606404

[9] Boursinos LA, Karachalios T, Poultsides L, Malizos KN. Do steroids, conventional non-steroidal anti-inflammatory drugs and selective Cox-2 inhibitors adversely affect fracture healing? J Musculoskelet Neuronal Interact. 2009; 9(1):44–52

[10] Koh W, Nguyen KP, Jahr JS. Intravenous non-opioid analgesia for peri- and postoperative pain management: a scientific review of intravenous acetaminophen and ibuprofen. Korean J Anesthesiol. 2015; 68(1):3–12

[11] Reuben SS. Effect of nonsteroidal anti-inflammatory drugs on osteogenesis and spinal fusion. Reg Anesth Pain Med. 2001; 26(6):590–591

[12] Karachalios T, Boursinos L, Poultsides L, Khaldi L, Malizos KN. The effects of the short-term administration of low therapeutic doses of anti-COX-2 agents on the healing of fractures. An experimental study in rabbits. J Bone Joint Surg Br. 2007; 89 (9):1253–1260

[13] Gajraj NM. The effect of cyclooxygenase-2 inhibitors on bone healing. Reg Anesth Pain Med. 2003; 28(5):456–465

[14] Sucato DJ, Lovejoy JF, Agrawal S, Elerson E, Nelson T, McClung A. Postoperative ketorolac does not predispose to pseudoarthrosis following posterior spinal fusion and instrumentation for adolescent idiopathic scoliosis. Spine. 2008; 33(10):1119–1124

[15] Horn PL, Wrona S, Beebe AC, Klamar JE. A retrospective quality improvement study of ketorolac use following spinal fusion in pediatric patients. Orthop Nurs. 2010; 29(5):342–343

[16] Glassman SD, Rose SM, Dimar JR, Puno RM, Campbell MJ, Johnson JR. The effect of postoperative nonsteroidal anti-inflammatory drug administration on spinal fusion. Spine. 1998; 23(7):834–838

[17] Dimar JR, II, Ante WA, Zhang YP, Glassman SD. The effects of nonsteroidal anti-inflammatory drugs on posterior spinal fusions in the rat. Spine. 1996; 21(16):1870–1876

[18] Park S-Y, Moon S-H, Park M-S, Oh K-S, Lee H-M. The effects of ketorolac injected via patient controlled analgesia postoperatively on spinal fusion. Yonsei Med J. 2005; 46(2):245–251

[19] Bergenstock M, Min W, Simon AM, Sabatino C, O'Connor JP. A comparison between the effects of acetaminophen and celecoxib on bone fracture healing in rats. J Orthop Trauma. 2005; 19 (10):717–723

[20] Smith AN, Hoefling VC. A retrospective analysis of intravenous acetaminophen use in spinal surgery patients. Pharm Pract (Granada). 2014; 12(3):417

[21] Cindea I, Balcan A, Gherghina V, et al. The impact of epidural analgesia on postoperative outcome after major abdominal surgery. In: Fyneface-Ogan S, ed. Epidural Analgesia: Current Views and Approaches. Rijeka, Croatia: InTech; 2012

[22] Mann C, Pouzeratte Y, Boccara G, et al. Comparison of intravenous or epidural patient-controlled analgesia in the elderly after major abdominal surgery. Anesthesiology. 2000; 92(2):433–441

[23] Ezhevskaya AA, Mlyavykh SG, Anderson DG. Effects of continuous epidural anesthesia and postoperative epidural analgesia on pain management and stress response in patients undergoing major spinal surgery. Spine. 2013; 38(15):1324–1330

[24] Guilfoyle MR, Mannion RJ, Mitchell P, Thomson S. Epidural fentanyl for postoperative analgesia after lumbar canal decompression: a randomized controlled trial. Spine J. 2012; 12(8):646–651

[25] Choi S, Rampersaud YR, Chan VWS, et al. The addition of epidural local anesthetic to systemic multimodal analgesia following lumbar spinal fusion: a randomized controlled trial. Can J Anaesth. 2014; 61(4):330–339

[26] Fisher CG, Belanger L, Gofton EG, et al. Prospective randomized clinical trial comparing patient-controlled intravenous analgesia with patient-controlled epidural analgesia after lumbar spinal fusion. Spine. 2003; 28(8):739–743

[27] Schenk MR, Putzier M, Kügler B, et al. Postoperative analgesia after major spine surgery: patient-controlled epidural analgesia versus patient-controlled intravenous analgesia. Anesth Analg. 2006; 103(5):1311–1317

[28] Gessler F, Mutlak H, Tizi K, et al. Postoperative patient-controlled epidural analgesia in patients with spondylodiscitis and posterior spinal fusion surgery. J Neurosurg Spine. 2016; 24(6):965–970

[29] Kluba T, Hofmann F, Bredanger S, Blumenstock G, Niemeyer T. Efficacy of post-operative analgesia after posterior lumbar instrumented fusion for degenerative disc disease: a prospective randomized comparison of epidural catheter and intravenous administration of analgesics. Orthop Rev (Pavia). 2010; 2(1):e9

[30] Christie IW, McCabe S. Major complications of epidural analgesia after surgery: results of a six-year survey. Anaesthesia. 2007; 62(4):335–341

[31] Black S. Postoperative analgesia after major spine surgery: patient-controlled epidural analgesia versus patient-controlled intravenous analgesia. Pain Manage. 2008; 2008:116–117

[32] Horan TC, Culver DH, Gaynes RP, Jarvis WR, Edwards JR, Reid CR, National Nosocomial Infections Surveillance (NNIS) System. Nosocomial infections in surgical patients in the United States, January 1986-June 1992. Infect Control Hosp Epidemiol. 1993; 14(2):73–80

[33] Shiono Y, Watanabe K, Hosogane N, et al. Sterility of posterior elements of the spine in posterior correction surgery. Spine. 2012; 37(6):523–526

[34] Veeravagu A, Patil CG, Lad SP, Boakye M. Risk factors for postoperative spinal wound infections after spinal decompression and fusion surgeries. Spine. 2009; 34(17):1869–1872

[35] Wimmer C, Gluch H, Franzreb M, Ogon M. Predisposing factors for infection in spine surgery: a survey of 850 spinal procedures. J Spinal Disord. 1998; 11(2):124–128

[36] Boody BS, Jenkins TJ, Hashmi SZ, Hsu WK, Patel AA, Savage JW. Surgical site infections in spinal surgery. J Spinal Disord Tech. 2015; 28(10):352–362

[37] Tomov M, Mitsunaga L, Durbin-Johnson B, Nallur D, Roberto R. Reducing surgical site infection in spinal surgery with betadine irrigation and intra-wound vancomycin powder. Spine. 2015; 40 (7):491–499

[38] Menekse G, Kuscu F, Suntur BM, et al. Evaluation of the time-dependent contamination of spinal implants: prospective randomized trial. Spine. 2015; 40(16):1247–1251

[39] Sweet FA, Roh M, Sliva C. Intrawound application of vancomycin for prophylaxis in instrumented thoracolumbar fusions: efficacy, drug levels, and patient outcomes. Spine. 2011; 36(24):2084–2088

[40] Molinari RW, Khera OA, Molinari WJ, III. Prophylactic intraoperative powdered vancomycin and postoperative deep spinal wound infection: 1,512 consecutive surgical cases over a 6-year period. Eur Spine J. 2012; 21(4) Suppl 4:S476–S482

[41] Lu S, Ma SC, Wang YY, Zhu ZH, Fan HW, Zhao GQ. Comparison of pain relief between patient-

controlled epidural analgesia and patient-controlled intravenous analgesia for patients undergoing spinal fusion surgeries. Arch Orthop Trauma Surg. 2015; 135(9):1247–1255

[42] Liu N, Wood KB, Schwab JH, et al. Comparison of intrawound vancomycin utility in posterior instrumented spine surgeries between patients with tumor and nontumor patients. Spine. 2015; 40(20):1586–1592

[43] Evaniew N, Khan M, Drew B, Peterson D, Bhandari M, Ghert M. Intrawound vancomycin to prevent infections after spine surgery: a systematic review and meta-analysis. Eur Spine J. 2015; 24(3):533–542

[44] Martin JR, Adogwa O, Brown CR, et al. Experience with intrawound vancomycin powder for spinal deformity surgery. Spine. 2014; 39(2):177–184

[45] Iwata E, Shigematsu H, Koizumi M, et al. Lymphocyte count at 4 days postoperatively and CRP level at 7 days postoperatively. Spine. 2016; 41(14):1173–1178

[46] Inanami H, Oshima Y, Iwahori T, Takano Y, Koga H, Iwai H. Role of 18F-fluoro-D-deoxyglucose PET/CT in diagnosing surgical site infection after spine surgery with instrumentation. Spine. 2015; 40(2):109–113

[47] Ahmed R, Greenlee JD, Traynelis VC. Preservation of spinal instrumentation after development of postoperative bacterial infections in patients undergoing spinal arthrodesis. J Spinal Disord Tech. 2012; 25(6):299–302

[48] Collins I, Wilson-MacDonald J, Chami G, et al. The diagnosis and management of infection following instrumented spinal fusion. Eur Spine J. 2008; 17(3):445–450

[49] Hedequist D, Haugen A, Hresko T, Emans J. Failure of attempted implant retention in spinal deformity delayed surgical site infections. Spine. 2009; 34(1):60–64

[50] Onen MR, Yuvruk E, Karagoz G, Naderi S. Efficiency of hyperbaric oxygen therapy in iatrogenic spinal infections. Spine. 2015; 40(22):1743–1748

10 Surgical Situations of Complex Decision-Making

Abstract

In the SFC approach to PDLS surgery, the surgeon assesses each patient as an individual case, factoring in the many clinical factors, and the radiographic presentation, in the attempt to make the appropriate therapeutic decision. The formulation of this decision can be complex in common scenarios.

Patients often present with incapacitating claudication from stenosis at a level with degenerative spondylolisthesis. The decision for, or against, adjunctive stabilization at the time of decompression requires an evaluation for antigravity axial pain, and a thorough assessment of radiographic features. A significant number of these patients are stable; others are clearly not so, requiring stabilization. In those patients with radiographic ambiguity as to stability, the individual clinical features must have greater directive force for the surgeon.

Sagittal alignment should be assessed in patients requiring multi-level decompression for stenosis, as significant SIB may predispose for poor outcomes secondary to low back pain. T1 pelvic axis (TPA) may be the best measure in this assessment. The decision for/against stabilization is relative to the extent of TPA abnormality and to individual clinical factors.

Frequently, the PDLS surgeon is presented with a patient having chronic progressive incapacitating anti-gravity axial pain. The decision for therapeutic arthrodesis can be a difficult one, especially when there are multiple degenerative levels. In this situation, there is no present diagnostic capacity able to differentiate the pain-generator level. When there are one or two degenerative levels, then surgery can be considered, but only when a thorough clinical and radiographic evaluation reveals certain features.

Keywords: lumbar stenosis, spondylolisthesis, Modic 1 changes, chronic axial lumbar pain, anti-gravity, sagittal imbalance, sagittal alignment

Whoever thinks a faultless piece to see,
Thinks what never was, nor is, nor ever shall be.

Alexander Pope

10.1 Lumbar Stenosis with Degenerative Spondylolisthesis (L3–L4 or L4–L5): Fusion or Not

10.1.1 Introduction

Symptomatic lumbar stenosis is commonly found with degenerative spondylolisthesis (DS) at the affected level. This stenosis most frequently results in primary radicular claudication involving the traversing root(s). There may be a chronic axial lumbar pain (CALP) component but this axial pain is likely related to underlying degenerative disc/interspace pathology. Spondylolisthesis is relatively prevalent and does not, of itself, contribute directly to lumbar pain either with or without spondylolysis.[1]

The degenerative chronic axial lumbar pain, when coexistent with radicular pain, is most frequently *antigravity pain (CALPag)* to be distinguished from the sometimes para-axial lumbar pain (unilateral or bilateral) seen in stenosis induced by walking/standing, with or without overt LE (lower extremity) claudication (and may represent dorsal rami symptomatology).

DS *can be stable*[2] and stabilization may not be required in selected patients.[3] Computed tomography (CT) scans may indicate arthrodesis in over 20% of cases, and such spontaneous fusion may be the common end-stage result in most instances.[4] The

129

surgeon who is faced with decompression for stenosis, in the DS setting, must decide the likelihood of DS progression postoperatively, with potential recurrence of radicular symptoms. It must be acknowledged that noninstrumented decompression has the highest rate of survival without eventual need for secondary surgery when it can be done without significant risk for progressive slip.[5] The specific decompression technique may be factorial for this progression.[6] Furthermore, and as expected, decompression without fusion is significantly more cost effective.[7]

A degeneratively fused segmental listhesis would need no prophylactic stabilization assuming judicious surgical removal of the posterior stability architecture. However, in the absence of such radiographic (CT) evidence of arthrodesis, the surgeon must rely on radiographic and clinical evidence of current "instability" though this term has not been clearly defined in this setting. *The decision to fuse or not is multifactorial and individualized. The recommendations for fusion below are conservative, with other authors suggesting lower threshold for stabilization especially in regard to definition of translational instability.*[8]

10.1.2 Image Evaluation

- CT scan:
  - Evidence of facet fusion.
  - Lateral and/or anterior osteophytes.
  - Interspace: anterior elevation ("fish-mouthing"), parallel, anterior collapse.
- Magnetic resonance imaging (MRI) scan:
  - Stenosis.
  - Facet gapping = size of facet effusion[9] and size/shape and angle of facet orientation.
  - Degree of anterolisthesis in the supine position.
  - Modic changes.
- Standing lateral lumbar radiographs with flexion[10]:
  - Progression of listhesis from the supine position (MRI or CT scan) to the standing position.

- Increased translation in the flexed position.
- Rotation degree at the level of listhesis.
- Bone quality.
- Radiographic sagittal alignment (SA) evaluation:
  - Sagittal vertical axis (SVA) and T1 pelvic axis (TPA); pelvic incidence-lumbar lordosis differential (PI-LL).
  - If listhesis is "fish-mouthed," then measurement of degree (vs. parallel endplates).

10.1.3 Physical Examination

- Flexing/erecting: grade level of *antigravity pain.*
- Size/habitus of patient.

10.1.4 Stability of Spondylolisthesis[11]

- CT evidence of stabilization: facet arthrodesis, disc height loss, fused bridging osteophytes, end plate sclerosis, ossification of anterior or posterior disc/ligament complex.
- No induced translational slip greater than 3 mm.
- No abnormal disc angle change with standing or flexion (physiologic rotation).
- Low grade antigravity pain (grade 0 or 1).

10.1.5 Major Indications for Consideration of Fusion

- Induced translational slip of greater than 3 mm and/or MRI facet effusion > 3.5 mm.[12]
- Rotational disc angle change resulting in loss of anterior disc height of at least 50%.
- Axial antigravity pain of at least grade 3.

10.1.6 Relative Indications for Consideration of Fusions

- Measurable but less than 3 mm of induced translational slip (especially at L4–L5).[8]

- Obesity (BMI [body mass index] > 40).
- At level of the DS, maintained disc height (greater than 10 mm).[13]
- Axial antigravity pain of grade 2 with Modic I changes.
- Any facet effusion (T2 enhancement on MRI).

10.1.7 Technical Considerations in Fusion

- Reduction is rarely necessary (with decompression) and can be detrimental.[14]
- Consideration of sagittal imbalance (SIB) as a causative factor.
- If interspace is "fish-mouthed" (representing bilateral pars defects), this may represent stress response to a preslip SIB and so interbody spacer and/or reduction may reduce its lordotic benefit (and throw patient back into a SIB).
- It is not necessary to extend an L4–L5 fusion to the sacrum when there is degenerative disc disease at L5–S1.[15]
- Noninstrumented fusion (with autograft) may be warranted in cases of osteoporosis or small pedicles.
- In a large retrospective cohort analysis, noninstrumented and instrumented fusions have been shown to have similar long-term complication and reoperation rates (with decreased costs of noninstrumentation).[16]
- In the acute postoperative phase, posterolateral fusion (PLF) alone has reduced complications and length of stay/charges compared to PLF in combination with interbody placement.[17]

10.2 Lumbar Stenosis with Severe Sagittal Imbalance: Sagittal Correction or Not

10.2.1 Introduction

As stated earlier, sagittal alignment (SA) parameters must be given consideration whenever the surgeon anticipates the need for fusion. Patients with lumbar stenosis should also have sagittal parameters evaluated. Patients with neurogenic claudication will compensate by reducing their LL in order to increase ambulatory comfort. This may cause characteristic gate when the patient leans forward with flexed knees. Such standing posture will obviously distort SA parameters often resulting in measured SIB. With surgical decompression, there will be an improvement in the reactively diminished lumbar lordosis and SA as the patient can resume normal lordotic posture of the lumbar spine without pain.[18,19] These studies suggested that both the LL and the TK (thoracic kyphosis) curves increase after decompression. The LL curves increased to a greater extent with positive net effect on SA, depending on the number of levels decompressed: 3 to 4 degrees with one to two levels and 6 to 7 degrees with three to four levels.

In the place of SVA preoperatively, the measurement of TPA may prove to be a better preoperative measurement assessing the underlying intrinsic sagittal alignment and thus the need for correction beyond that provided by laminectomy alone. As the TPA is independent of pelvic compensation mechanisms (i.e., retroversion), any net corrective effect (LL-TK) will be reflected directly and proportionally in the TPA. However, the use of TPA in this setting is not as yet confirmed.

As SIB can be an independent factor for LBP,[20] residual SIB (> 50 mm) after lumbar decompression for stenosis would be expected to yield inferior results, especially in regard to pain and functional measurement. This has been shown to be the case and a delineation of preoperative SA > 80 mm (severe SIB) portends this possibility.[21] However, studies attributing postoperative LBP to SIB must take into account other LBP etiologies unaffected by sagittal balance. These possibilities would include residual radicular pain and/or degenerative discogenic pain.[22]

10.2.2 Image Evaluation

The evaluation of neurogenic claudication from lumbar stenosis should include the following.

- MRI scan:
  - Number of levels (including potential remote development).
  - Central (hypertrophic ligamentum flavum) versus lateral recess stenosis.
- Radiologic SA evaluation/compensation:
  - SVA, PI-LL, TPA.
  - Sacrofemoral axis (as evidence for hip flexion).
  - PT (pelvic tilt), PS (pelvic shift), KFA (knee flexion angle).
- Plain X-rays:
  - AP (anteroposterior)/lateral L spines.
  - Standing flexion/extension laterals.
  - Hip X-rays (as necessary per examination).

10.2.3 Physical Examination

- Reflex asymmetry; unanticipated presence/extent of reflexes (suggesting possibility of concurrent cervical stenosis/myelopathy).
- Supine evaluation for flexion–contracture at the hip (attempt to lie flat with knees unflexed and heels on the surface); Thomas' maneuver.
- Flexion and re-erection for antigravity pain.

10.2.4 Published Recommendations for Consideration of Need for Sagittal Correction

- SVA > 80.[21]
- PI-LL > 21.5 and SVA > 69.[18]

10.2.5 Suggested Recommendations Using TPA

- Goal: establishment of post-op TPA of < 10.
- Measurement of pre-op TPA:
  - If < 20: minimal potential for problematic post-op SIB and/or LBP.
  - If 20–25 (marginal imbalance): consider sagittal correction if one or two levels of decompression is needed; if three or four levels of decompression is needed, then follow up TPA (with back pain symptoms).
  - If > 25: individualized consideration for sagittal correction.

10.3 Severe Antigravity Chronic Axial Lumbar Pain: To Fuse or Not

The evidence for the efficacy of fusion for "CLBP" is conflicting and there remain more questions than answers.[23] "CLBP" is a heterogenous condition[24] and this issue will not be resolved without the formulation of a clear definition and a standardized clinical subclassification system, as discussed earlier. Without subgroup analysis, any therapeutic evaluation is limited. One extensive clinical study on three randomized controlled trials (RCTs) acknowledged this limitation, yet noted that the data suggested that surgical treatment had "… a greater proportion of very good and very poor outcomes … than with non-operative care." Thus, the imperative is to establish which patients have a "very good" response, and why.

Unfortunately, the research paradigm of RCTs has not changed much in the last 20 years. And as one extensive review has stated: "Rather than clarifying what, if any, indications for surgery exist, investigators in the field continue to analyze variations in surgical technique, which will probably have very little impact on patient outcomes."[25]

A recent systematic review and meta-analysis of all RCTs on "discogenic" LBP to date suggests that both operative treatment and nonoperative management/PT are "… acceptable treatment methods for intractable LBP."[26] But the selection criteria across the studies were inconsistent and heterogenous, clinically and radiographically. Thus, there is no clinical relevance for the surgeon in the evaluation of the individual patient in this or other such meta-analyses.

Those studies that are positive for fusion are often directed at "discogenic" LBP[27,28, 29,30]; but this term is not consistently defined. It is well known that degenerative radiographic markers (high-intensity zones [HIZ], Modic changes,[31,32] disc morphology, osteophytic changes) have little overall predictive value for the development, extent, or localization of pain generator in CLBP.[33] There are reports attempting to establish the relevance of more specific features of these (e.g., Modic type)[34] signal intensities of HIZ[35] or of a calculated combination of morphologic features (MRI index)[36] to be used as a biomarker to identify the pain generator. Of these markers, Modic I changes may be most consistently associated with active CLBP.[37] However, Modic I changes have been shown to progress to a more stable Modic II in the majority of patients (though not all) over the course of 1 to 5 years,[38] which may be a function of increase in stability.[39] Furthermore, Modic I changes have been shown to revert to normal.[40] All of these studies, however, relate to a clinically *nonspecific* CLBP.

Provocative discography has been called the "gold standard" in the determination of "discogenic" back pain and its use has been shown to have considerable influence on surgical decision-making.[41] But discography remains controversial. Diagnostic discoblock (interspace anesthetic) has been reported as being a valuable guide in providing a strict diagnosis of discogenic back pain. In one report, limited to patients with one-level disease, the use of discoblock in addition to provocative discography defined candidates for fusion that had significant postoperative improvement versus a minimal treatment control group.[42] A small randomized study suggested that discoblock is a useful tool for diagnosis of discogenic LBP as compared to discography.[27]

Without more specificity, it is inappropriate to consider fusion surgery for a heterogenous and poorly defined pain condition (i.e., "CLBP") based solely on degenerative radiographic features. The surgical decision for fusion (below) is based on a more specific definition of chronic pain in the lower back, confirmed by a long-standing history and examination, with a specific radiologic (MRI) appearance. Such a selective approach seems reasonable at the present level of understanding. Subclassification of chronic pain in the lower back will allow for greater investigational specificity, eventually yielding a more accurate selection process with avoidance of negative responders.

10.3.1 Relative Indications for Fusion in Chronic Axial Lumbar Pain, Antigravity Type (CALPag)

- History:
  - Pain progressive for at least 2 years without totally pain-free periods.
  - Pain with or without acute onset.
  - Pain is functionally incapacitating; described as severe in "getting up and down"; patient admits to difficulty getting things off floor: done by spouse or

133

children; has long-handled grasper or avoids attempts altogether.

o Hip/leg symptoms, if present, are secondary.

o Psychosocial distress is identified and deemed appropriately treated.

- Alternative therapies ineffective:
  o Patient has participated in McKenzie/MDT (mechanical diagnosis and therapy) evaluation and therapy and/or cognitive/behavioral therapy, which have been ineffective.[43,44]
  o Injections: ESIs (epidural steroid injections); facet.
  o Modic antibiotic spine therapy (MAST; with severe Modic I changes)[45,46]: investigational.

- Physical examination:
  o Precise axial (midline) localization of primary point of pain (PPP).
  o Focal tenderness with spinous process pressure in prone position, with or without palpable fasciculations.
  o Grade 3 or 4 antigravity pain with flexion/re-erection.

- MRI scan (positive surgical indication features):
  o Index single severe degenerative level corresponding to PPP with no more than one other (lesser) degenerative level.
  o Modic I changes at the index level.
  o Bone marrow edema (via gadolinium-enhanced via coronal T1 and/or T2 fat-saturated images).[47]
  o Deformity: anterolisthesis and/or lateral listhesis.

- Discogram (optional):
  o Severe annular disruption at index level, with concordant pain.

- *Plain radiographs* with standing flexion/extension laterals and scoliosis surgery (**for surgical technique direction**):
  o Note translational listhesis standing greater than supine (i.e., MRI) and flexion/extension excursion.
  o Note measures of SIB: SVA, TPA, and LL-PI.

10.4 Unknowns and Investigational Opportunities

- Further refinement of the radiographic definition of translational (sagittal) "instability" or definition of absolute stability.
- Further investigation into the role of regional/global SA in outcomes with noninstrumented decompressions.
- Definition of pain generator in chronic axial antigravity lumbar pain (CALPag).
- Role of MAST therapy in treatment of CALPag.
- Role of bone marrow edema (vs. Modic I changes) as directive of surgical therapy of CALPag.

References

[1] Kalichman L, Kim DH, Li L, Guermazi A, Berkin V, Hunter DJ. Spondylolysis and spondylolisthesis: prevalence and association with low back pain in the adult community-based population. Spine. 2009; 34(2):199–205

[2] Hasegawa K, Kitahara K, Shimoda H, et al. Lumbar degenerative spondylolisthesis is not always unstable: clinicobiomechanical evidence. Spine. 2014; 39(26):2127–2135

[3] Joaquim AF, Milano JB, Ghizoni E, Patel AA. Is there a role for decompression alone for treating symptomatic degenerative lumbar spondylolisthesis? Clin Spine Surg. 2016; 29(5):191–202

[4] Huang KT, Adogwa O, Babu R, Lad SP, Bagley CA, Gottfried ON. Radiological evidence of spontaneous spinal arthrodesis in patients with lower lumbar spondylolisthesis. Spine. 2014; 39(8):656–663

[5] Brodke DS, Annis P, Lawrence BD, Woodbury AM, Daubs MD. Reoperation and revision rates of 3 surgical treatment methods for lumbar stenosis associated with degenerative scoliosis and spondylolisthesis. Spine. 2013; 38(26):2287–2294

[6] Chang HS, Fujisawa N, Tsuchiya T, Oya S, Matsui T. Degenerative spondylolisthesis does not affect the outcome of unilateral laminotomy with bilateral decompression in patients with lumbar stenosis. Spine. 2014; 39(5):400–408

[7] Kim S, Mortaz Hedjri S, Coyte PC, Rampersaud YR. Cost-utility of lumbar decompression with or without fusion for patients with symptomatic

degenerative lumbar spondylolisthesis. Spine J. 2012; 12(1):44–54

[8] Jang J-W, Park J-H, Hyun SJ, Rhim S-C. Clinical outcomes and radiologic changes after microsurgical bilateral decompression by a unilateral approach in patients with lumbar spinal stenosis and grade I spondylolisthesis with a minimum 3-year follow-up. Clin Spine Surg. 2016; 29(7):268–271

[9] Ben-Galim P, Reitman CA. The distended facet sign: an indicator of position-dependent spinal stenosis and degenerative spondylolisthesis. Spine J. 2007; 7(2):245–248

[10] Segebarth B, Kurd MF, Haug PH, Davis R. Routine upright imaging for evaluating degenerative lumbar stenosis. J Spinal Disord Tech. 2015; 28 (10):394–397

[11] Simmonds AM, Rampersaud YR, Dvorak MF, Dea N, Melnyk AD, Fisher CG. Defining the inherent stability of degenerative spondylolisthesis: a systematic review. J Neurosurg Spine. 2015; 23 (2):178–189

[12] Kuhns B, Kouk S, Buchanan CC, et al. Sensitivity of MRI in the diagnosis of L4–5 degenerative Spondylolisthesis. Spine J. 2014; 14(11):S61

[13] Sato S, Yagi M, Machida M, et al. Reoperation rate and risk factors of elective spinal surgery for degenerative spondylolisthesis: minimum 5-year follow-up. Spine J. 2015; 15(7):1536–1544

[14] Lian X-F, Hou T-S, Xu J-G, et al. Posterior lumbar interbody fusion for aged patients with degenerative spondylolisthesis: is intentional surgical reduction essential? Spine J. 2013; 13(10):1183–1189

[15] Liao J-C, Chen W-J, Chen L-H, Niu C-C, Keorochana G. Surgical outcomes of degenerative spondylolisthesis with L5-S1 disc degeneration: comparison between lumbar floating fusion and lumbosacral fusion at a minimum 5-year follow-up. Spine. 2011; 36(19):1600–1607

[16] Lad SP, Babu R, Ugiliweneza B, Patil CG, Boakye M. Surgery for spinal stenosis: long-term reoperation rates, health care cost, and impact of instrumentation. Spine. 2014; 39(12):978–987

[17] Norton RP, Bianco K, Klifto C, Errico TJ, Bendo JA. Degenerative Spondylolisthesis. Spine. 2015; 40 (15):1219–1227

[18] Fujii K, Kawamura N, Ikegami M, Niitsuma G, Kunogi J. Radiological improvements in global sagittal alignment after lumbar decompression without fusion. Spine. 2015; 40(10):703–709

[19] Jeon C-H, Lee H-D, Lee Y-S, Seo H-S, Chung N-S. Change in sagittal profiles after decompressive laminectomy in patients with lumbar spinal canal stenosis: a 2-year preliminary report. Spine. 2015; 40(5):E279–E285

[20] Jackson R, Behee K, McManus A. 5. Sagittal spinopelvic alignments standing and in an intraoperative prone position. Spine J. 2004; 4(5):S5

[21] Hikata T, Watanabe K, Fujita N, et al. Impact of sagittal spinopelvic alignment on clinical outcomes after decompression surgery for lumbar

spinal canal stenosis without coronal imbalance. J Neurosurg Spine. 2015; 23(4):451–458

[22] Bayerl SH, Pöhlmann F, Finger T, et al. The sagittal balance does not influence the 1 year clinical outcome of patients with lumbar spinal stenosis without obvious instability after microsurgical decompression. Spine. 2015; 40(13):1014–1021

[23] Deyo RA. Fusion surgery for lumbar degenerative disc disease: still more questions than answers. Spine J. 2015; 15(2):272–274

[24] Fourney DR, Andersson G, Arnold PM, et al. Chronic low back pain: a heterogeneous condition with challenges for an evidence-based approach. Spine. 2011; 36(21) Suppl:S1–S9

[25] Andrade NS, Flynn JP, Bartanusz V. Twenty-year perspective of randomized controlled trials for surgery of chronic nonspecific low back pain: citation bias and tangential knowledge. Spine J. 2013; 13(11):1698–1704

[26] Bydon M, De la Garza-Ramos R, Macki M, Baker A, Gokaslan AK, Bydon A. Lumbar fusion versus nonoperative management for treatment of discogenic low back pain: a systematic review and meta-analysis of randomized controlled trials. J Spinal Disord Tech. 2014; 27(5):297–304

[27] Ohtori S, Kinoshita T, Yamashita M, et al. Results of surgery for discogenic low back pain: a randomized study using discography versus discoblock for diagnosis. Spine. 2009; 34 (13):1345–1348

[28] Ohtori S, Koshi T, Yamashita M, et al. Existence of pyogenic spondylitis in Modic type 1 change without other signs of infection: 2-year follow-up. Eur Spine J. 2010; 19(7):1200–1205

[29] Pekkanen L, Neva MH, Kautiainen H, Kyrölä K, Marttinen I, Häkkinen A. Changes in health utility, disability, and health-related quality of life in patients after spinal fusion: a 2-year follow-up study. Spine. 2014; 39(25):2108–2114

[30] Phillips FM, Slosar PJ, Youssef JA, Andersson G, Papatheofanis F. Lumbar spine fusion for chronic low back pain due to degenerative disc disease: a systematic review. Spine. 2013; 38(7):E409–E422

[31] Modic MT, Steinberg PM, Ross JS, Masaryk TJ, Carter JR. Degenerative disk disease: assessment of changes in vertebral body marrow with MR imaging. Radiology. 1988; 166(1, Pt 1):193–199

[32] Jensen TS, Karppinen J, Sorensen JS, Niinimäki J, Leboeuf-Yde C. Vertebral endplate signal changes (Modic change): a systematic literature review of prevalence and association with non-specific low back pain. Eur Spine J. 2008; 17(11):1407–1422

[33] Kalichman L, Kim DH, Li L, Guermazi A, Hunter DJ. Computed tomography-evaluated features of spinal degeneration: prevalence, intercorrelation, and association with self-reported low back pain. Spine J. 2010; 10(3):200–208

[34] Kaapa E, Luoma K, Pitkaniemi J, Kerttula L, Grönblad M. Correlation of size and type of Modic types 1 and 2 lesions with clinical

symptoms: a descriptive study in a subgroup of patients with chronic low back pain on the basis of a university hospital patient sample. Spine. 2012; 37(2):134–139

[35] Liu C, Cai H-X, Zhang J-F, Ma JJ, Lu YJ, Fan SW. Quantitative estimation of the high-intensity zone in the lumbar spine: comparison between the symptomatic and asymptomatic population. Spine J. 2014; 14(3):391–396

[36] Bechara BP, Agarwal V, Boardman J, et al. Correlation of pain with objective quantification of magnetic resonance images in older adults with chronic low back pain. Spine. 2014; 39(6):469–475

[37] Järvinen J, Karppinen J, Niinimäki J, et al. Association between changes in lumbar Modic changes and low back symptoms over a two-year period. BMC Musculoskelet Disord. 2015; 16(1):98

[38] Rahme R, Moussa R. The Modic vertebral endplate and marrow changes: pathologic significance and relation to low back pain and segmental instability of the lumbar spine. AJNR Am J Neuroradiol. 2008; 29(5):838–842

[39] Lao L, Daubs MD, Scott TP, et al. Effect of disc degeneration on lumbar segmental mobility analyzed by kinetic magnetic resonance imaging. Spine. 2015; 40(5):316–322

[40] Hutton MJ, Bayer JH, Powell JM. Modic vertebral body changes: the natural history as assessed by consecutive magnetic resonance imaging. Spine. 2011; 36(26):2304–2307

[41] Berg S, Isberg B, Josephson A, Fällman M. The impact of discography on the surgical decision in patients with chronic low back pain. Spine J. 2012; 12(4):283–291

[42] Ohtori S, Koshi T, Yamashita M, et al. Surgical versus nonsurgical treatment of selected patients with discogenic low back pain: a small-sized randomized trial. Spine. 2011; 36(5):347–354

[43] Mannion AF, Brox JI, Fairbank JCT. Comparison of spinal fusion and nonoperative treatment in patients with chronic low back pain: long-term follow-up of three randomized controlled trials. Spine J. 2013; 13(11):1438–1448

[44] Dufour N, Thamsborg G, Oefeldt A, Lundsgaard C, Stender S. Treatment of chronic low back pain: a randomized, clinical trial comparing group-based multidisciplinary biopsychosocial rehabilitation and intensive individual therapist-assisted back muscle strengthening exercises. Spine. 2010; 35(5):469–476

[45] Albert HB, Sorensen JS, Christensen BS, Manniche C. Antibiotic treatment in patients with chronic low back pain and vertebral bone edema (Modic type 1 changes): a double-blind randomized clinical controlled trial of efficacy. Eur Spine J. 2013; 22(4):697–707

[46] Albert HB, Kjaer P, Jensen TS, Sorensen JS, Bendix T, Manniche C. Modic changes, possible causes and relation to low back pain. Med Hypotheses. 2008; 70(2):361–368

[47] Nakamae T, Yamada K, Shimbo T, et al. Bone marrow edema and low back pain in elderly generative lumbar scoliosis. Spine. 2016; 41(10):885–892

11 Socioeconomics in Spine Surgery

Abstract

The huge increase in national healthcare expense has resulted in the interjection of economic "stakeholders" into the medical decision processes. Cost-effectiveness (CE) analysis, utilizing comparative effectiveness research (CER), has established the cost/QALY value metric, based on utility health-related quality of life (HRQL) outcome measures. There are unavoidable limitations in the establishment of this metric.

These administrative/political cost-control initiatives have increasingly relied on evidence-based medicine (EBM), primarily generated by medical science investigation. Randomized controlled trials (RCTs) are considered the gold standard of investigational studies, though other forms of study are valid. RCTs and their systemic reviews via meta-analysis give averaged data; they can be definitive or non-definitive and may fail to account for outlier results. The use of EBM data to the PDLS surgeon often is limited within the setting of the examining room. Over-reliance on such data can have detrimental effects on the patient-care process.

The rise of surgical spine-care expense has outpaced that of the general national healthcare. This is primarily the result of the increasing use of instrumentation [for fusion]. Instrumentation/fusion technology has benefitted many patients. However, the multibillion dollar industry of its use has corrupted the process establishing clinical indications and efficacy. This has been done mainly by incorporating the surgeon into the corporate profit stream, establishing significant conflict of interest (COI) scenarios within product investigational research.

The fundamental solution to the exponential rise in over-all healthcare expense entails the conversion of its economic model into one that establishes a diagnostic unit of purchase, as apposed to the present interventional one. And in spinal surgery, the instrumentation/fusion industry must be removed, financially, from the process of product investigation and validation.

Keywords: cost-effectiveness, comparative effectiveness research, cost/QALY, randomized controlled trials, evidence-based medicine, conflict of interest, , , ,

There can be no liberty unless there is economic liberty.

Margaret Thatcher

11.1 Introduction

In the last two decades, the expense of surgical spine care has risen dramatically, and at a higher rate than other inpatient procedures.[1] The number of lumbar fusions increased 2.7-fold between 1998 and 2008. The overall national spending for spinal fusion increased from \$4.3 billion to \$33.9 billion in this period. This trend has not abated in the 7 years since, and does not translate into improved health status. The fact that, nationally, surgical spine care costs are rising at a pace greater than that of overall surgical health care expenditure suggests unique economic features within this subspecialty.

Economic "stakeholders" have assumed a greater scrutiny of the medical decision processes. Cost-effectiveness (CE) analysis has established methods used in comparative effectiveness research (CER). CER has been defined by the Institute of Medicine as "… the generation and synthesis of evidence that compares the benefits and harms of alternative methods to prevent, diagnose, treat and monitor a clinical condition or to improve the delivery of care. The purpose of CER is to assist consumers, clinicians, purchasers, and policy makers to make informed decisions that will improve health care at both the individual and population levels."[2]

CER has developed equations for using outcome-based investigational studies in establishing relative interventional **value** (see next section). **Evidenced-based medicine (EBM)**, therefore, has assumed a greater relevance in times of unsustainable increases in health care expenditures. Investigational studies have always been a part of valid scientific inquiry and method to inform the practicing medical clinician, the emphasis being on establishing improved methods of care and ruling out potentially harmful ones. The introduction of value measurement has qualified the clinician's use of investigational results by imposing an economic rationale in interventional decision-making.

Establishing valid investigational outcome comparisons in the interventional care of the painful degenerative lumbar spine (PDLS) is extremely challenging (see below). This difficulty has been in part the consequence of inherent clinical factors: the extreme diversity of individual pathology, the variance of medical status of study subjects rendering poor control of potential response factors, and the subjective nature of these outcome responses. Besides problematic issues in outcome measurement, investigational design may have poor control over standardization of the intervention studied. A multicenter study, for example, may involve surgeons with differing educations, training, experience, and technical capability.

11.2 Cost/ Quality-Adjusted Life Years: Metric of Relative interventional Value

Value is defined as directly proportional to quality and inversely so to cost. The standard economic formula is therefore $V = Q/C$.

If quality is established as a measurable entity, then cost effectiveness (CE) may be defined as the inverse of the value equation: $CE = cost/measured\ quality$.

Quality is established by outcome measurement. Presently, various types of health-related quality of life (HRQL) measures are used in spine care evaluation. *Patient-centered* measures are preferable in value establishment, and include the following:

- Disease-specific measures, e.g., Oswestry Disability Index (ODI) and Neck Disability Index.
- General health-related outcome measures, e.g., SF-36 (36-Item Short Form Survey) and derivatives/versions (SF-12, SF-8, SF-6D).
- Utility measures[3] are based on economic and decision theory requiring patient to establish a subjective point of indifference between two health conditions, e.g., Euroqol EQ-5D, Health Utility Index, SF-6D (derived from SF-36 and SF-12)

Concept of "QALY" (quality adjusted life years): a calculated measure that incorporates a time-length factor for an established outcome-based quality measurement. *Utility* outcome measures are used in QALY computation, though there is a conversion formula relating ODI to SF-6D and thus making ODI usable in QALY calculation.

Cost measurement is complicated and without a standard method of calculation. Both "direct" and "indirect" costs are included.

- Direct costs: those attributable to actual patient care. Complexity of calculation secondary to lack of "price" transparency and their variances, and the reliance on patient recall.
- Indirect costs: those attributable to lack of productivity. Calculation with time factor is not standardized and often requires patient-reported data.

Cost/QALY: a standard monetary **value** metric of an intervention as established by outcome-based quality assessment with limitations of calculation complexity, non-uniformity, and patient recall in data collection.

11.3 Evidence-based Medicine

11.3.1 Defined

The other major initiative in the control of health care costs, one mainly directed by medical professionals, is the thrust toward establishing establishing evidence-based medicine (EBM). EBM has become the catch phrase for evaluating the relationship between clinical application and scientific validity. It has been defined as "... the use of mathematical estimates of the risk of benefit and harm, derived from high-quality research on population samples, to inform the clinical decision-making in the diagnosis, investigation or management of individual patients."[4,5] As noted earlier, this definition could be expanded, since EBM outcome data inform economic as well as clinical decision-making.

There are several forms of primary studies, all of which can have EBM validity in various situations. *Cohort studies* require long-term follow-up (sometimes decades) when two groups have had different exposures to a health-altering agent (including a defined surgical procedure). *Case control studies* usually address rare conditions and involve retrospective investigation of diseased and control groups in order to establish potential etiological factors. *Cross-sectional surveys* are often run by epidemiologists who collect specific data (related to medical care) from a representative sample at a single time point. *Case reports and case series* are generally considered as relatively weak as scientific evidence, but there are "...good theoretical grounds for the reinstatement of the humble case report as a useful and valid contribution to medical science, not the least because the story is one of the best vehicles for making sense of a complex clinical situation."[6]

11.4 Randomized Controlled Trials: Limitations for the PDLS Surgeon

Randomized controlled trials (RCTs) are the gold standard for investigational studies establishing *therapeutic* guidance. They are considered at the pinnacle of the hierarchy of medical evidence informing clinical decision-making. However, the statistical significance of an RCT may be "fragile," meaning a small number of outcome events can eliminate significance.[7] And not all RCTs are "high-quality research"; some are patently invalid.

RCTs present averaged ("population") data that are often of marginal benefit in the examining room, wherein the PDLS surgeon is interacting with the individual patient presenting with a pain complaint (which may or may not be of spinal etiology). The value of RCTs in degenerative spine surgery is further limited by nonuniform application of the investigated therapy, by large variability in comorbid substrate, and by subjectivity of outcome reporting. The swallowing of a pill is essentially the same by all subjects in a drug trial. On the other hand, lumbar fusion as a therapeutic measure will have a multitude of variances that can affect the individualized result: specificity of indication, procedural type and technique, experience of surgeon, patient comorbidities and psychosocial state, in-hospital and postoperative care, etc. And in a drug trial, the outcome data are usually reported as a distinct, objective, and measurable quantity. Fusion surgery outcome measurement, conversely, may have one or more of many different forms (functional, quality of life pain scales), all of which are more qualitative and subjective.

Statistically, higher investigational numbers provide greater interpretive accuracy in measurement of therapeutic outcome. Hence, the results of *systematic reviews* of RCTs with *meta-analysis* of data can have greater practical relevance for the degenerative spine surgeon. However, the individual RCTs incorporated in these reviews have great heterogeneity in study design. And these RCTs can have limited application due to exclusion criteria, inclusion bias, disregard of qualitative aspects, publication bias, conflict-of-interest (COI) effects, inappropriate statistical evaluation, and accuracy.[8,9] Many of these deficiencies are unavoidably transmitted to these large database studies and their incorporation will cause distortion of conclusions. Furthermore, clinical significance and statistical significance are not necessarily the same.[10]

Thus for the degenerative spine surgeon, literature review often provides confusing guidance, if any at all, for the treatment of the individual patient with a pain complaint referable to the degenerative spine. In a systemic review, the surgeon may encounter an *averaged* conclusion that may or may not support a particular therapeutic effort. This surgeon will also likely discover that investigational results data will present some very positive individual outcomes and some poor ones. *Such a spectrum of outcome is consequent to a fundamental complexity of evaluation and surgical decision-making in surgery for the PDLS.* The degree of this complexity has a direct relationship to the extent of positive and negative **outliers.**

As a conceptual example, the efficacy of lumbar fusion for axial back pain may be investigated, versus nonoperative treatment as in the clinical study by Mannion et al.[11] Such a reported systematic review of the literature may have no supportive evidence, or only weak evidence, for such

surgery. And yet there will be certain individual cases of undeniable and dramatic success within the results data. The surgeon will note that the systemic review addressed surgical therapeutic outcome as measured in subjects with "chronic low back pain" (CLBP). There was no subclassification of this amorphous symptom according to its cause of onset, its course, its precise location/radiation, its relation to activity, etc. Thus, the conclusion of the systemic review was based on an averaged surgical therapeutic response for a nonspecific symptomatic entity. Any potential benefit of fusion for a more specifically defined subform of chronic back pain is obscured within the systemic review.

Should a study or studies report fusion results with more target specificity, there may be a different conclusion as to the efficacy of surgical fusion therapy. If, for instance, the "CLBP" studied was precisely subdefined as *lumbar axial* (centered midline), as *specific to activity causation* (antigravity elevation), and was *coexistent with particular radiographic abnormality* (marked interspace changes predominant at one level), then lumbar fusion for this subset of patients with "CLBP" may be validated as EBM.

In the earlier example, the genesis of the concept of a possible relationship between efficacy of lumbar fusion and a more specific subdefinition of "CLBP" can emerge only from clinical experience. The practicing physician/surgeon that is involved in the evaluation and treatment of degenerative spine pain provides the conceptual substrate for investigational studies. *Thus, better care of patients with PDLS, surgical or nonsurgical, is primarily engendered by an interactive symptom-focused experience between the clinician and the individual patient.*

11.5 Conclusion

- Surgical spine care costs are increasing in an unsustainable manner and various "stakeholders" initiatives have developed accordingly.

- Economic "stakeholders" have established the methods of CER, which uses economic mathematical tools to measure the relative *monetary value* in health care *interventions.*
- Cost/QALY is a standard metric of relative interventional value and uses *utility* investigational outcomes in quality assessment.
- Medical professionals have concentrated on the concept of EBM to measure *clinical value* in health care interventions by investigational literature evaluation.

EBM conclusion is dependent on the quality of studies investigated.

- RCTs and their systemic reviews (with meta-analysis of their data) are considered at the top of the hierarchy informing clinical decision-making. Thus, EBM uses these studies as the predominant form for investigational evaluation though other types of investigational literature may have considerable value, including case reports.
- RCTs can have definitive or nondefinitive results as defined by whether or not confidence intervals overlap the *threshold of clinically significant effect.*[6]
- The complexities in the surgical care of the PDLS often limit the clinical application of EBM because of averaging of group data. And EBM has practical, philosophical, and ethical limitations.[12,13]

11.5.1 Potential Detrimental Effects of EBM

- Undermines therapeutic management strategy at the individualized patient level.[14]
- Is a value given undue importance relative to professional experience.[15]
- Is used as a clinical directive based on evaluation of studies of poor quality, by design, method, and/or statistical evaluation.

- Is a clinical directive corrupted by COI within the studies investigated or by the review EBM author(s) (see next section).
- Results in a conclusion that obscures the need for population subset investigation.
- Is used by health care purse holders to deny coverage for positive outlier individuals.

Symptom-focused clinical care provides the conceptual basis for investigative initiatives into interventional therapeutic effectiveness with special applicability in surgery on the PDLS.

11.6 Economics and Ethics in Spine Surgery: The Perfect Storm

The human spirit must prevail over technology.

Albert Einstein

The explosive increase in the expense of the surgical care of the spine, from 1998 to 2008, has been discussed earlier. That trend has not abated in the 7 years since. Also, as mentioned, this exponential increase has exceeded that of the general rise in overall health care expenditure. Thus, there are unique features to spine surgery, within this time frame, that must account for such discrepancy. Yet any discussion as to the process for addressing this unsustainable trend in spine surgery must necessarily engage the general economic health care environment in the United States.

11.6.1 Fundamental Causes of the Rise in Expense of Surgical Spine Care

- *A health care system functioning without market controls.* The present health care economic system is essentially a *cost-driven system.* Economic transactions are not subject to price/value competition. Attempts to bring costs into a competitive market framework have involved some form of their "bundling"[16] into price-like entities that have had limited competitive effect. The main thrust of cost control therefore has been in the realm of *care control* through CE analysis and emphasis on the directives of EBM as noted in the previous section. At the fundamental level, these are initiatives to control how the practicing physician makes medical interventional decisions. But they will remain relatively ineffectual as long as the *health care unit of purchase is an intervention.*

- **Health care reimbursement on the basis of intervention.** Health care is delivered as a *service.* Market competition in financial transaction based on service provision (vs. sale of *goods*) is more subject *to incentive* manipulation. Service provided at an hourly rate, for instance, has competitive value as it allows for one provider's rate to be compared with that of the other. But once a provider is chosen, there is no control on how *financially efficient* (ultimate expense) that service is provided. Inherently, there will be a negative incentive for expediency as payment for that service is directly proportional to the time it takes to provide it. *But should reimbursement for that service be a predetermined amount, then such negative incentive for financial efficiency is removed and is replaced by positive productivity incentive.*

An informative analogy can be taken from the legal profession, with regard to the expense for a *defined service.* The payment for an attorney's production of a contract can be based on an hourly rate, which is neither financially nor productively efficient because of a negative financial incentive for quick completion. Should the cost of contract production be a *predetermined amount* (as indeed it used to be), then the

effective efficiency incentive consequence is positive.

Furthermore, not only does a *predetermined price* for a *defined service* align incentive toward production efficiency, and away from financial inefficiency, but it also has real **market-competitive value**, if that price is openly set by, or agreed to, by the provider.

The challenge in health care expense, therefore, is to establish a reimbursement system that pays a *predetermined price* for a *defined service.* Health care reimbursement currently is based on *interventional purchase units, i.e., defined service = (an) intervention.* Cost-reduction stakeholders, therefore, have attempted to establish *predetermined price per intervention.* And payers have used their purse-holder leverage to exact such *intervention-price agreement* from providers. But an *intervention*-based payment system is similar incentively to the one based on hourly rates, in that the more interventional steps taken, the greater the reimbursement. Provider incentive in an *intervention*-based payment system is thus negative for financial efficiency. Expense control by *intervention pricing* is limited to the extent that there is control over the *number of interventions.* Consequently, there are evermore attempts by payers to limit this number by precertification obfuscation, denials based on reliance of averaged scientific data, demands of different (less expensive) *interventions*, etc. *At this point, health care decisions have moved from the professional provider to the payer/administrator.*

The solution (discussed later) is to disequate *intervention* from *defined service.* In the legal analogy, the appropriate *defined service* would be the produced contract. As noted, this *defined service* is incentive positive and market competitive. But if the defined service in this legal analogy was, instead, the production of a paragraph or other textual subunit of the completed contract, then these advantages are lost.

Similarly, in health care when *intervention* is the *defined service*, incentives are undermined and market-competitive value is lost. The forces of expense containment can then only rely on forced *intervention* pricing and care-control measures of limiting *intervention* numbers.

If incentive and market competition are to be inherent expense-control mechanisms in health care, then the *defined service* cannot be an *intervention*. Rather, it must be reestablished into some other form of *defined product*.

- **The advent of instrumentation/products in spinal surgical care.** Instrumentation/fusion in spinal surgical care has become a multibillion dollar industry. This is represented by multiple profit centers per every surgical instrumentation case: the hardware and its application tools, bone fusion products, graft-harvesting equipment, radiographic technology, cell-saving (blood conservation) machines, neuromonitoring abilities, etc. There have been huge conglomerate corporations built around this industry and hundreds of companies involved in some smaller niches—all pushing the case for their product.

These products add a huge expense to spinal surgery. Furthermore, their surgical use often requires a much more extensive surgery with intendant increase in OR (operating room)/anesthesia expense, greater complication rate (and the expense to deal with them), more rehabilitative and home health care expense, later return to work, etc.

To be sure, instrumentation and other surgical products have improved the care of many patients and continue to do so. However, the consequence of adverse incentives by surgeons (and other providers) has often clouded the validity of the indication and effectiveness of their use. Though this resulting corruptive influence in spinal surgery has been noted for years,[17] it continues enhanced and unabated.

The adverse incentive has two forms. The first is more general and is directly related to the *intervention*-based reimbursement system as discussed earlier. As surgical charges are based accordingly, larger surgeries result in *more interventions* and thus potentially greater remuneration for the surgeon. And, the *intervention*-based charges are often very large. Hence, in any given case, the surgeon has financial incentive to do an extensive procedure. Within the present environment, the professional ethic provides the dominant restraint on the abuse of this system, but unfortunately, this ethic is succumbing to the power of money. Hence, exogenous care-control measures (as discussed earlier) are increasing to stem potential overuse of these products.

It is extremely important to note that such overuse may exist not as a cognitive volitional act by the surgeon, but rather as the consequence of a subtle but cogent change of mindset engendered by a surgical science that has been adulterated by the economics of the surgical products industry.

The mechanism by which this industry has subverted surgical science is through their *incorporation of the provider as a financial beneficiary, directly or indirectly.* Hence, the second form of adverse incentive by the provider is specific to this relationship.

- *Incorporation of the surgeon (other providers) as financial beneficiaries of product success.* There are several ways by which surgeons can benefit financially by product success. Intellectual property (IP) ownership is legitimate and sometimes hugely lucrative. Such opportunity has spawned hundreds of new spine surgery–related patents. However, the establishment and publication of the clinical validity of these products is rarely independent. It is common that the patent holder and/or manufacturer of a new product either underwrites or manages such investigation. An industry employee can be a principal investigator without repercussion as an unacceptable bias.

The surgical literature is replete with extensive COI disclosures by authors. Besides patent/royalty declaration, other financially beneficial relationships with the product industry is protean and commonplace: ongoing consultancies, stock and stock option ownership, research support, travel expenses to training venue (often exotic), seminar support and recompensation, corporate board membership, etc. Disclosure requirement is now mandatory by most publications. However, transparency does not absolve of bias. "It cannot be overemphasized that most effects of any bias induced by COIs are unconscious, partly instinctive, partly psychological and almost always unintentional."[18]

Research support by industry has been lauded and encouraged. When such grants support the investigation of a product with financial ramification for the supporting company and/or researchers, prejudice is unavoidable. Such studies may be presented as high-value RCTs, yet this bias can be obscured within in multiple ways. The surgeon in general clinical practice rarely has the time, or the methodological and statistical knowledge, for an accurate analysis of the scientific validity of these articles aside from the reported conclusions. Thus, there are internal and external limitations to accountability in industry-supported research.

In conclusion, industry techniques of integrating corporate financial interest with that of the surgeon have contributed to the explosive increase in use of fusion-related instrumentation and products. There is inherent potential bias in industry-supported research into the clinical validity of instrumentation/products when study investigators have direct or indirect financial interest in product success. This "marketing disguised as research"[19] can be blatantly absurd and dangerous.[20] Most often, however, the bias is subtly persuasive and difficult to detect. *And, importantly, conclusions reported in abstracts are* *discrepant with the full manuscript in a high proportion of published articles.*[21]

11.6.2 Fundamental Solution: From Cost Driven to Price Controlled

- **Change the unit of health care purchase (reimbursement) from *intervention* to *diagnosis*.** A diagnostic-based unit would be defined with symptoms and/or pathology. Such unit prices would be *predetermined.* Its establishment would allow for comparative value assessment and thus would be *market competitive*. It could also be used to give competitive value across surgical specialties (see below).

A significant advantage of the diagnostic-based pricing unit would be its effect on provider (surgeon's) evaluative technique and operative plan. The surgeon's interaction with the patient would necessarily be aligned with an explicit understanding of the patient's primary complaint and the precise etiology thereof. Radiographic/MRI (magnetic resonance imaging) presentation would have secondary etiological relevance as revealing abnormality congruent to patient symptomatology. This refocus on patient presentation, as directed by the *diagnostic reimbursement unit*, will cause a needed shift of the evaluative surgeon's mindset away from one concerned primarily with radiographic abnormality and its instrumented correction.

Incentive realignment follows. If the surgeon is receiving one reimbursement price for operative correction of the established diagnosis, the incentive will be to do so in the most limited way possible (i.e., as symptom-focused care). The operative plan would be closely linked to the established diagnosis. Any decision to use instrumentation, for example, will be supported, and mandated, by the clinical diagnosis. *Precertification by purse holders would be addressed to the clarification of diagnosis rather than to the operative plan.*

The established operative diagnoses can be tiered. As an example, surgery for the PDLS might include as an elementary (but instructive) example:

- *Class 1:* Discogenic/stenotic root compression with unilateral or bilateral symptoms, at single vertebral level.
- *Class 2:* Discogenic/stenotic root compression with unilateral or bilateral symptoms, at two vertebral levels.
- *Class 3:* Discogenic/stenotic root compression with unilateral or bilateral symptoms at more than two vertebral levels.
- Class 4:
  1. Lumbar instability at one vertebral level, with axial antigravity pain and/or radicular symptoms, requiring one-level stabilization.
  2. Severe (grade 3–4) chronic axial antigravity lumbar pain (CALPag) from degenerative disc disease, one vertebral level, requiring one-level arthrodesis for pain control.
- *Class 5:* As per class 4 but with the requirement of two-level stabilization/arthrodesis.
- Class 6: As per class 4 (1) but with requirement of three levels of stabilization.
- Class 7: As per class 4 (2) but with requirement of more than three levels of stabilization.

Hence reimbursement for all such surgeries on the PDLS will be at one of six prices. (This is in contrast to the present system where reimbursement involves hundreds of codes and modifiers that require specially trained coding personnel for appropriate compliance.)

The *competitive value* of these prices can extend beyond spine surgery if similar hierarchies are established in other surgical specialties, and thus the price of a specific class in one specialty can be compared to that of the same class in another specialty.

In a true free-market system, these prices would be openly established by the provider giving the payor(s) expense with which to make value comparison. And, importantly, the expense is predetermined and as such there would be accountability for any deviance. Surgical billing would become transparent.

- **Prohibition of COI in research.** Authors of published research literature should have no financial stake in the outcome of medical/surgical research. The effects of the *Physician Payments Sunshine Act* have been minimal. It is well documented that, otherwise, *bias is unavoidable despite disclosure requirements*, specifically in regard to surgical instrumentation/products:
  o Their investigation should not include any author who is a patent holder or who potentially will receive royalties or any other direct or indirect income from the use or sale of investigated product.
  o Their investigation should not include any author with any *ongoing* financial relationship with the product manufacturer/developer such as in direct employment, consultancy, board membership, etc.

It should be noted that the North American Spine Society (NASS) Professional Recommendations suggest that industry support of clinical and basic science research is acceptable as long as data analysis is uninfluenced by sponsors, and second-party objective external data analysis is strongly encouraged.[22] However, in regard to investigation involving instrumentation/product evaluation, the study design, methods, and data collection can all reflect bias if the investigators have financial interest in the study results. Furthermore, the NASS position holds that COI does not necessarily equate to bias. This is, to some degree, in contradistinction to an article published in their front-line socioeconomic publication.[18]

- **Prohibition of COI in marketing and/or education**. Any surgeon who has any financial stake in the success of a product, or a financial relationship with its manufacturer/developer, should be prevented in its marketing and education to other providers. That surgeon should not be allowed to host any seminar or course related to the application of such product; nor should the venue for such be at that surgeon's institution. That surgeon should be allowed no payment/stipend other than as per any other attendee.
- **Prohibition of industry support of medical education.** "The responsibility for medical education should be entirely in the hands of the medical profession and funding should not compromise, or even call into question, the integrity and independence of what is taught or of the physicians who teach."[23]

References

[1] Rajaee SS, Bae HW, Kanim LE, Delamarter RB. Spinal fusion in the United States: analysis of trends from 1998 to 2008. Spine. 2012; 37(1):67–76

[2] Gogawala Z, Resnick DK. Comparative effectiveness research: what does this mean for spine care in the United States. SpineLine. 2011; 12(2):20–23

[3] Rihn J, Currier B, Prather H. Measuring outcomes and value in spine care. SpineLine. 2011:25–30

[4] Greenhalgh T. How to Read a Paper: The Basics of Evidence-Based Medicine. 5th ed. New York, NY: John Wiley & Sons; 2014

[5] Greenhalgh T. How to Read a Paper: The Basics of Evidence-Based Medicine. 5th ed. New York, NY: John Wiley & Sons; 2014:1

[6] Greenhalgh T. How to Read a Paper: The Basics of Evidence-Based Medicine. 5th ed. New York, NY: John Wiley & Sons; 2014:38–41

[7] Evaniew N, Files C, Smith C, et al. The fragility of statistically significant findings from randomized trials in spine surgery: a systematic survey. Spine J. 2015; 15(10):2188–2197

[8] Yoshihara H, Yoneoka D. Understanding the statistics and limitations of large database analyses. Spine. 2014; 39(16):1311–1312

[9] Greenhalgh T. How to Read a Paper: The Basics of Evidence-Based Medicine. 5th ed. New York, NY: John Wiley & Sons; 2014:34–38

[10] Maltenfort MG. Understanding large database studies. J Spinal Disord Tech. 2015; 28(6):221

[11] Mannion AF, Brox JI, Fairbank JCT. Comparison of spinal fusion and nonoperative treatment in patients with chronic low back pain: long-term follow-up of three randomized controlled trials. Spine J. 2013; 13(11):1438–1448

[12] Tonelli MR. The philosophical limits of evidence-based medicine. Acad Med. 1998; 73(12):1234–1240

[13] Straus SE, McAlister FA. Evidence-based medicine: a commentary on common criticisms. CMAJ. 2000; 163(7):837–841

[14] McGirt M. Measuring value of spine care at the individual patient level. SpineLine. 2014; 15 (6):26–29

[15] Watters WC, III. Ethical decision making: the physician-patient relationship. SpineLine. 2014; 15(1):8–9

[16] Sharan A. A systems approach to managing the delivery of healthcare. SpineLine.. 2016; 17(1):19

[17] Robertson JT. The rape of the spine. Surg Neurol. 1993; 39(1):5–12

[18] Schofferman J. Conflicts of interest: biological and psychological mechanisms of bias. SpineLine. 2012; 13(2):37–39

[19] Rosen CD. It's not about the money. Spine J. 2011; 11(8):700–702

[20] Carragee EJ, Hurwitz EL, Weiner BK. A critical review of recombinant human bone morphogenetic protein-2 trials in spinal surgery: emerging safety concerns and lessons learned. Spine J. 2011; 11(6):471–491

[21] Lehmen JA, Deering RM, Simpson AK, Carrier CS, Bono CM. Inconsistencies between abstracts and manuscripts in published studies about lumbar spine surgery. Spine. 2014; 39(10):841–845

[22] Wetzel FT. A primer of industry relationships with spine care professionals & professional associations (PMA). SpineLIne. 2014; 15(2):33–35

[23] Relman AS. Industry support of medical education. JAMA. 2008; 300(9):1071–1073

Index

A

A-delta fibers 30
ABI (ankle-brachial index) 58
acetaminophen 133
adjacent segment disease (ASD)
- indications for stabilization 33, 50
- junctional kyphosis and 44
- pathophysiology 44
adult degenerative scoliosis (ADS)
- sagittal balance evaluation, pre-operative 41
- surgery for, vs. SFC surgery for PDLS 48
--coronal deformity imperatives 50
--image evaluation 49
--patient presentation 49
--sagittal balance imperatives 49
affect 66
anatomy, fundamentals of, see specific structures
- muscular 16
- neurological 26
- overview 15
- pelvis 34
- skeletal 18
- space definitions 15
- unknowns and investigational opportunities 31
ankle-brachial index (ABI) 58
anterior plexus 27
antibiotic prophylaxis 107, 122, 135
antigravity/mechanical chronic axial lumbar pain (CALPag), see chronic axial lumbar pain (CALP)
area of pain 60
arthrodesis 43–44
ascending pain pathways 30

B

bacterial infections 62
Beck Depression Inventory (BDI) 67
behavioral assessment 65
biomechanics, lumbar degenerative changes and 44
bleeding, in MIS fusion 122
bone healing, NSAIDs and 133
bone morphogenetic protein (BMP) 123

C

C fibers 30
C-reactive protein and postoperative infection 136
cage migration, prevention of 122
CALP, see chronic axial lumbar pain (CALP)
case control studies 149
case reports (case series) 149
Castellvi radiography classification system 23, 25
center of mass and gravity line 35
central stenosis 53
CER (comparative effectiveness research) 147–148
cerebrospinal fluid leakage 107
chronic axial lumbar pain (CALP)
- antigravity/mechanical (CALPag) 61
- clinical evaluation 61
--grading scale for 61
--indications for fusion 143
--pathophysiology 61
--stabilization procedures 50
--surgical decision-making 71
- compression-loading (CALPcl) 61, 71
- possible infectious etiology 62
- randomized controlled trials, operative vs. nonoperative treatment 142
- surgical decision-making process 71, 142
chronic pain predominant in lower back 59
- See also sacroiliac joint pain
- clinical evaluation 60
--historical points 60
--physical examination 61, 62
- precise clinical description of lower back pain 60
circumferential plexus 27
CLBP (chronic low back pain), see chronic pain predominant in lower back
clinical evaluation, PDLS 53
- chronic axial pain of lumbar spine, possible infectious etiology 62
- chronic pain predominant in lower back 59
- neurogenic pain in hip and leg 53
- nonneurogenic leg pain 57
- nonradicular neurogenic leg pain syndromes 55
- overview 53
- psychosocial factors 65
- radicular pain 54
- sacroiliac joint pain 63

unknowns and investigational opportunities 67
clinical trials, see randomized controlled trials (RTCs)
cognitive/behavioral factors, in surgical outcome 66
cohort studies 149
common peroneal nerve, neuropathy of 57
comparative effectiveness research (CER) 147–148
compensatory mechanisms, sagittal imbalance 36, 36
complications, see specific surgical procedures
- minimally invasive surgery
--decompression 107
--lumbar interbody fusion 122
- sacroiliac joint fusion 65
- surgical decision-making, open vs. MIS surgery 104
compression-loading chronic axial lumbar pain (CALPcl) 61, 71
cone of balance 35, 38
conflict of interest
- health care costs and 154
- prohibiting in marketing and education 156
- prohibiting in research 155
conjoined nerve root 27
coronal deformities 47
coronal plane metrics 41
coronal scoliosis 50
cost effectiveness analysis 147
Cox (nonselective cyclooxygenase) inhibitors 132–133
cross-decompression, bilateral 77, 79
cross-sectional surveys 149
crying, in clinical evaluation 67

D

decision-making, surgical
- complex decision-making
--lumbar stenosis with degenerative spondylolisthesis, fusion or not 139
--lumbar stenosis with severe sagittal imbalance, sagittal correction or not 141
--severe antigravity chronic axial lumbar pain, fusion or not 142
--situations requiring 139
- open vs. minimally invasive surgery 104

– operative plan with primary axial low back pain 71
– operative plan with radicular pain presentation 71
– psychosocial factors 65
– unknowns and investigational opportunities 144
decompression with nonoperated anatomy
– minimally invasive surgery 105
– open surgery 72
decompression, bilateral
– cross-decompression 77, 79
– dual-tube medial foraminotomy (MIS) *109*, 109
– unilateral single-tube laminectomy 111, *112*
– with U-Turn and contralateral decompression 75, *79*
decompressive surgery, symptom-focused care and 13
– *See also* minimally invasive surgery (MIS), open surgical methods
degenerative hip disease 58
– examination 59
– hip joint innervation and 58
– investigation of 59
– lumbar stenosis vs. 58
– pain history and 59
– treatment 59
depression and surgical prognosis 66
diagnosis in symptom-focused care 12–13
diclofenac 133
disability application, questioning about 67
discectomy
– far lateral nerve root decompression (MIS) 114, *115*
– medial, unilateral decompression of nerve root 106, 107, *108–109*
– minimally invasive 103
discogenic pain 54
discography, provocative 143
Distress and Risk Assessment Method (DRAM) 67
dorsal nerve root 26
dorsal ramus 26, 28
dorsal root ganglion 26
drug abuse 67
dural penetration 122
dural tears 107–108, 122
durotomy, incidental 93, *96–97*

E

EBM, *see* evidence-based medicine (EBM)

endolac 133
entrapment neuropathies 56
– common peroneal nerve 57
– lateral femoral cutaneous nerve 56
– superior cluneal nerve 57
epidural access, alternative process of gaining 74, *76–78*
epidural analgesia, postoperative, *see* postoperative care (PEA)
ethics, medical
– economics and 151
– in symptom-focused care 13
evidence-based medicine (EBM)
– health cost controls and 148, 149
– measuring clinical value of interventions 151
– potential detrimental effects 151
– primary studies, forms of 149
– randomized controlled trials and 149
extensor muscle pathology 46
extraforaminal space 16
extreme lumbar interbody fusion (XLIF) *126*, 126

F

FABER test (bent-knee thigh rotation) 59
facet (zygapophyseal) joints 19
– architecture of 20
– destabilization and loss of functional integrity
––bilateral facet joint destabilization 20, *22*
––inferior articular process 20, *21*
––ipsilateral pars and contralateral lamina 20, *22*
––ipsilateral pars and ipsilateral lamina 20, *21*
– functional integrity 19
– intact, as operative landmarks to lateral corridor 19, *20*
fentanyl 134
foramen 15, *16*
foraminal space 16
foraminotomy
– dual-tube medial foraminotomy (bilateral decompression) *109*, 109
– unilateral decompression of nerve root with 106, 107, *108–109*
fusion techniques, minimally invasive 118
– *See also* lumbar interbody fusion, minimally invasive

G

gabapentin 132–133
gate control theory of pain 30, *31*
global coronal alignment 41
gravitational force, in lumbar degenerative changes 43
gravity line and center of mass 35
gray rami communicantes (GRCs) 27

H

health-related quality of life (HRQL) measures 148
hemilaminectomy 70, 83
herniation, *see* lumbar disc herniation
hip and leg pain, neurogenic vs. radicular 53
hip contracture, Thomas test for 59
hip flexion contracture 46
hip joint osteoarthritis, lumbar stenosis vs. 58
histrionics on examination 67

I

ibuprofen 133
iliac screws placement, S2 alar 89, *91*, 95
iliocostalis lumborum 28
iliolumbar ligament 23
indomethacin 133
infection control 135
– antibiotic prophylaxis 107, 122, 135
– deep space infection 136
– intrawound antibiotic powder 135
– operative techniques minimizing infection rate 135
– postoperative systemic markers 135
– risk factors 135
innervation 28
– intervertebral disks 29
– investigational opportunities 32
– skin 28–29
– spinal musculature 28
insomnia 67
interbody cages 14
intervertebral disks, innervation 29
intracanalicular space 16
intraforaminal space 16
intramuscular plane, lateral 17, *19*
intraspinous muscle, innervation 28
isthmic spondylolisthesis, 23

J

joint capsule, anatomy of 21
junctional kyphosis 44, 45
junctional stress, postoperative 44

K

ketorolac 133

L

laminectomy
 – bilateral, midline approach
  (MIS) 116, 118
 – en bloc technique 80, 83–85
 – piecemeal rongeuring 77, 79, 81–
  82
 – unilateral single-tube bilateral
  decompression (MIS) 111, 112
lateral femoral cutaneous nerve 56
lateral intramuscular planar approach, L3 to sacrum 97
 – iliac graft harvest as extension
  of 99, 102–103
 – interbody spacer placement 99,
  101–102
 – introduction 97
 – operative technique 98, 99–100
lateral intramuscular plane 17, 19
lateral plexus 27
lateral recess 15
laterality of pain 60
leg pain syndromes, nonradicular
  neurogenic 55–56
leg pain, nonneurogenic 57–58
leg-length discrepancy 41, 47
ligaments 22
 – iliolumbar ligament 23
 – ligamentum flavum
 – –anatomy 22, 24
 – –preservation of 72, 105
 – –removal of 105
longissimus muscle, innervation 28
lordosis, lumbar (LL) 34, 37
low back pain, chronic (CLBP), see
  chronic pain predominant in lower back
lumbar degeneration, gravitational
  force in 43
lumbar disc herniation
 – as contraindication for MIS decompression 106, 109, 111, 127
 – bacterial infections and 63
 – cauda equina decompression
  and 116
 – conjoined nerve roots and 27
 – laminectomy with midline disc
  herniation 117

 – nerve root compression and 115
 – radicular pain and 14
lumbar interbody fusion, minimally
  invasive 118
 – approaches to 119, 119
 – complications 122
 – extreme (XLIF) 126, 126
 – introduction 118
 – posterior (PLIF) 123, 123
 – transforaminal 118, 120
lumbar lordosis (LL) 34, 37
lumbar pain and disability, sagittal
  misalignment in 33
lumbar plexus 26, 26
lumbar region, para-axial 55
lumbar stenosis
 – degenerative spondylolisthesis
  and 139
 – hip joint osteoarthritis vs. 58
 – radicular pain in 55
 – severe sagittal imbalance
  and 141
 – uncompensated sagittal imbalance and 46
lumbosacral plexus 26
lymphocyte count and postoperative
  infection 136

M

magnetic resonance imaging (MRI)
 – conjoined nerve root 27
 – patient examination and 13
 – radicular pain evaluation 54
market controls, lack of 152
medical education, prohibiting industry support of 156
meloxicam 133
meralgia paresthetica 56
midlumbar segmental deformity,
  surgical considerations 47
minimally invasive surgery (MIS)
 – advantages and disadvantages vs.
  open techniques 103, 128
 – decompression techniques 106
 – –bilateral decompression (dual-
  tube medial foraminotomy) 109,
  109
 – –complications 107
 – –far lateral nerve root decompression (lateral discectomy) 114,
  115
 – –laminectomy (bilateral, midline
  approach) 116, 118
 – –laminectomy (unilateral single-
  tube bilateral decompression) 111, 112
 – –unilateral decompression of nerve
  root 106, 108–109
 – –with nonoperated anatomy 105

 – fundamentals of 105
 – fusion techniques 118, 119
 – –complications 122
 – –extreme lumbar interbody fusion
  (XLIF) 126, 126
 – –posterior lumbar interbody fusion
  (PLIF) 123, 123
 – –transforaminal lumbar interbody
  fusion 118
 – introduction 102
 – lumbar spine surgery and future
  of 129
 – opening and closure of surgical
  incision 105
 – operative plan 104
 – SFC surgery and 14
Modic changes, chronic low back
  pain and 62, 143
Modified Somatic Perception Questionnaire (MSPQ) 67
Modified Zung Depression Index
  (mZDI) 67
mood and personality factors, in
  surgical outcome 66
multifidus muscle 16, 28
multimodal pain control, postoperative 132
multisegmental and migrating complaints 66
muscular anatomy 16
 – construction crane analogy 17
 – innervation 28
 – investigational opportunities 31
 – lateral intramuscular plane 17,
  19
 – multifidus 16
 – pars lumborum 17
 – pars thoracis 17

N

naproxen 133
nerve root compression 30, 31
nerve rootlets 26
neurogenic claudication 54, 141
neurogenic pain 53, 55
neurological anatomy 26
 – conjoined nerve roots 27
 – gate control theory of pain 30, 31
 – innervation 28
 – pain pathways 30
 – somatic nerves 26
 – sympathetic nerves 27
nociceptors 30
nonradicular leg pain syndromes 55
nonselective cyclooxygenase (Cox)
  inhibitors 132–133
nonsteroidal anti-inflammatory
  drugs (NSAIDs)
 – analgesia and 133

- bone healing and spinal fusion, effects on 133
- preemptive use of 132

O

obesity, multisegmental spondylosis and 36
open surgical methods 70
- advantages and disadvantages vs. MIS 103, 128
- decision-making processes 71
- decompression techniques
--bilateral decompression with U-Turn and contralateral decompression 75, 79
--cross-decompression, bilateral 77, 79
--root decompression 70
--root/dural decompression with joints intact 88, 89, 92–93
--U-Turn technique (unilateral decompression of nerve root with nonoperated anatomy) 72, 74–76
--with nonoperated anatomy 72
- epidural access, alternative process of gaining (best at L5ûS1) 74, 76–78
- extraforaminal root decompression
--via parsectomy 86, 86, 87
--with partial lateral parsectomy 87, 89–91
- fundamentals of 72
- hemilaminectomy 70, 83
- iliac screws placement, S2 alar 89, 91, 95
- incidental durotomy, repair and wound closure 93, 96–97
- introduction 70
- laminectomy 70
--en bloc technique 80, 83–85
--piecemeal rongeuring 77, 79, 81–82
- lateral intramuscular planar approach, L3 to sacrum 97
- pedicle screw placement, multistep process for 88, 93–94
- surgical incisions, opening and closure of 72, 73
operative landmarks to lateral corridor 18
- facet joint 19, 20
- spinous process/lamina 19, 20
Oswestry Disability Index (ODI) 148

P

pain control, postoperative

- epidural analgesia 134
- multimodal 132
- NSAIDs effect on bone healing 133
- systemic 132
pain pathways 30
- ascending 30
- descending 30
- investigational opportunities 32
painful degenerative lumbar spine (PDLS) surgery
- behavioral assessment 65
- clinical evaluation 53
- complex decision-making in 139
--See also decision-making, surgical
- minimally invasive surgical methods 101
--See also minimally invasive surgery (MIS)
- open surgical method, fundamentals of 70
--See also open surgical methods
- patient examination 12
- postoperative care 132
- socioeconomics 147
--See also socioeconomics in spine surgery
- symptom-focused care surgery 12
--adult degenerative scoliosis surgery vs. 48
--coronal deformity imperatives 49
--decompressive surgery and 13
--image evaluation 49
--patient presentation 49
--sagittal balance imperatives 49
--stabilization and 14, 43
paracetamol, see acetaminophen
pars lumborum 17
pars thoracis 17
patient examination 12
- image evaluation 13
- physical examination 13
- spinopelvic and global alignment 13
Patient Health Questionnaire Depression Module (PHQ-9) 67
Patient Reported Outcome Measurement Information System 67
patient-controlled IV analgesia (PCIA) 134
patient-surgeon interactions
- minimally invasive surgery 104
- open surgery decision-making 71
PDLS, see painful degenerative lumbar spine (PDLS) surgery
PEA (postoperative epidural analgesia) 134
pedicle screw (PS)

- compression of 122
- instrumentation 14
- multistep process for placement 88, 93–94
pelvic incidence (PI) 34, 36
pelvic obliquity 41, 47
pelvic shift 36, 36, 37
pelvic tilt (PT)
- equation for 35
- measurement of 35, 38
- uncompensated sagittal imbalance and 46
pelvis, anatomy of 34
physical examination 13
piroxicam 133
plumb-line variance 33
posterior lumbar interbody fusion (PLIF) 123, 123
posterior plexus 27–28
postoperative care 132
- about 132
- epidural analgesia (PEA) 134
--outcomes assessment 134
--patient-controlled, vs. patient-controlled IV analgesia 134, 134
--regimens and dosages 134
--techniques 134
- infection control 135
--See also infection control
- pain control, systemic 132
- unknowns and investigational opportunities 136
pregabalin 132–133
primary point of pain (PPP), localization of 60
projection neurons 30
Propionibacterium acnes 62
pseudoarthrosis 122
psychosocial factors
- behavioral assessment 65
- categories 66
- clinical evaluation techniques 66
- clinician-administered measurements 67
- formal assessment testing 67
- self-administered measurements 67
pyriformis syndrome 55
- history and diagnosis 56
- treatment 56

Q

quality adjusted life years (QALY) 148
quality of life measures, health-related (HRQL) 148

R

radiation of pain 60
radicular pain
– clinical evaluation 54
– discogenic vs. stenotic presentation 54, *55*
– historical points 54
– minimal examination for suspected root(s) involvement 54
– motor symptoms 54
– neurogenic pain vs., hip and leg 53
– operative plan, surgical decision-making 71
– presenting predominantly in lower back 55
––*See also* chronic pain predominant in lower back
– radiographic studies 54
– true radicular symptomology 54
randomized controlled trials (RTCs)
– limitations for PDLS surgeon 149
– operative vs. nonoperative treatment of CALP 142
– systematic reviews with meta-analysis 150–151
relative interventional value (cost/QALY) 148
risk factors, postoperative infection 135
root compression 47, 50
root decompression, extraforaminal
– via parsectomy 86, 86, *87*
– with partial lateral parsectomy 87, *89–91*
root/dural decompression with joints intact 88, *89, 92–93*
RTCs, *see* randomized controlled trials (RTCs)

S

sacral plexus 26, *26*
sacral slant (SS) 35, *36*
sacroiliac joint pain
– anesthetic block for diagnosing 65
– evaluation and surgical considerations 64
– injection therapy 64
– joint fusion for 65
– prevalence 63
sacroiliac joint, anatomy of 24
safe sublaminar space 16, *17, 23, 24*
sagittal alignment
– correlation with surgical outcomes 35, 47
– measurement of parameters 33, 47, *48*, 141

– pre-operative attention to 33
– surgical planning for correction of 46
sagittal balance 33
– *See also* sagittal imbalance, spinopelvic parameters
– center of mass and gravity line 35
– cone of balance 35, 38
– coronal plane metrics 41
– evaluation of 37
––fixed angular measurement, spine to pelvis 37
––global coronal alignment 41
––leg-length discrepancy 41
––pelvic incidence–lumbar lordosis (PI-LL) relationship 38, *41*
––pelvic obliquity 41
––plumb-lining measurement 37
––sagittal vertical axis (SVA) 37, *40*
––sagittal vertical axis and TPA vs. patient age 40
––spinopelvic inclination measurements 37
– introduction 33
sagittal imbalance (SIB)
– in patients not requiring stabilization 46
– limited stabilization role in SFC surgery 45, 50
– lumbar stenosis with, correction decision-making 141
––author's recommendations using TPA 142
––image evaluation 142
––physical examination 142
––published recommendations for sagittal correction 142
– outcome of multisegment decompression 34
– potential need for osteotomy 46
sagittal shoulder sign 27
sagittal tilt (ST) 39
sagittal vertical axis (SVA) 33, 37
SCID-1 (Structured Clinical Interview for DSM-IV Axis 1 Disorders) 67
scoliosis, coronal 50
– *See also* adult degenerative scoliosis (ADS)
SF-36 mental health scales 67
shoe string closure of dura 94, *96*
Short Form Health Survey (SF-36)
– as health-relate outcome measure 148
– mental health component 67
SIB, *see* sagittal imbalance (SIB)
side/symmetry of pain 60
sinuvertebral nerves 28

situational factors, in surgical outcome 66
skeletal anatomy 18
– facet architecture 20
– joint capsule 21
– ligaments 22
– lumbosacral transitional vertebrae 23
– operative landmarks to lateral corridor 18
– sacroiliac joint 24
– zygapophyseal (facet) joints 19
skin, innervation 28, *29*, 29
socioeconomics in spine surgery 147
– cost containment solutions
––competitive value of prices 155
––conflict of interest prohibitions 155–156
––diagnostic reimbursement unit 154
––incentive realignment 155
––industry support of medical education, prohibitions on 156
––tiered operative diagnoses 155
– evidence-based medicine and 149
––*See also* evidence-based medicine (EBM)
– increasing costs of spine surgery, causes of 152
––conflict of interest 154
––defined service vs. intervention reimbursement 152
––instrumentation and surgical products 153
––intervention-based health care reimbursement 152
––lack of market controls 152
––surgeons benefiting from product success 153
– introduction 147
– randomized controlled trials, limitations of 149
– relative interventional value 148
––cost/QALY metric 149
––quality adjusted life years 148
––quality measures 148
– research support by industry 154
– stakeholders in medical decision-making 147, 151
somatic nerves 26
– dorsal root ganglion 26
– lumbar plexus 26, *26*
– sacral plexus 26, 26
– spinal nerve 26
– sympathetic nerves interconnection with 27, *28*
spinal nerve 26
spinopelvic parameters 34

- *See also* sagittal balance
- lumbar lordosis (LL) 34, *37*
- pelvic incidence (PI) 34, *36*, 38
- pelvic incidence–lumbar lordosis (PI-LL) relationship 38, *41*
- pelvic tilt (PT) 35, *38*
- sacral slant (SS) 35, *36*
- sagittal tilt (ST) 39
- spinopelvic inclination, T1 and T9 37
- TI pelvic angle (TPA) 39, *41*, 141
spondylolisthesis
- adjunctive stabilization 14, 23
- degenerative, lumbar stenosis with 139
--image evaluation 140
--indications for considering fusion 140
--stability of spondylolisthesis 140
--technical considerations in fusion 141
spondylosis, multisegmental, obesity and 36
stabilization in SFC surgery 43
- adjunctive 14
- arthrodesis for 43
- coronal deformity considerations 50
- indications for segmental fusion/stabilization 50
- introduction 43
- negative consequences on sagittal alignment 47
- nonfusion techniques 43
- unknowns and investigational opportunities 51
Staphylococcus infections 62
stenosis, central 53
stenotic pain 54
Structured Clinical Interview for DSM-IV Axis 1 Disorders (SCID-1) 67

subarticular space 15
sublaminar space, safe 16, *17*, 23, *24*
substance abuse 67
substance P 30
superior cluneal nerve, neuropathy of 57
surgical incisions, opening and closure of
- minimally invasive surgery 105
- open surgery 72, *73*
surgical site infection, predictors of 135
sympathetic nerves 27
- circumferential plexus 27
- interconnection with somatic nerves 27, *28*
- sinuvertebral nerves 28
symptom-focused care (SFC), *see* painful degenerative lumbar spine (PDLS) surgery
- about 12
- definition 12
- description of pain 12
- diagnosis in 12–13
- ethical issues 13
- minimally invasive surgery 14
- patient examination 12
- psychosocial factors in surgical decision-making 65
systematic reviews with meta-analysis 150

T

Thomas test (hip contracture) 59
TI pelvic angle (TPA) 39, *41*, 141
transforaminal lumbar interbody fusion (TLIF) 118, *119*

U

U-Turn technique (unilateral decompression of nerve root with nonoperated anatomy) 73, *74–76*
unilateral decompression of nerve root
- with medial discectomy or foraminotomy 106, *108–109*
- with nonoperated anatomy 73, *74–76*

V

value, relative interventional (cost/QALY) 148
vancomycin powder 135
vascular claudication 57
- ankle-brachial index 58
- clinical evaluation 58
- history of 58
- treatment 58
ventral nerve root 26
ventral ramus
- anatomy 26
- skin innervation via *29*, 29

W

wrong side surgery 108

X

XLIF (extreme lumbar interbody fusion) *126*, 126

Z

Zung Depression Scale (ZDS) 67
zygapophyseal (facet) joints 19